Preface

The context of pre-hospital care is changing. Health organisations around the world are witnessing a strain on their operational budgets with increasing demand for their services. The pressures of ageing population, demographic changes, other socio-cultural factors and the changing role of the ambulance services in the wider health-care networks are all challenging the traditional model of ambulance delivery. This is further impacting on the effectiveness of the ambulance organisations and their responses to the various challenges discussed in this volume.

In addressing some of the key management themes, the volume relies upon a strong research base and critical insights. It brings together top quality scholarship using experts in their respective fields: academics, practitioners and professionals to each of the chosen topics. Our authors represent senior academics, chief executives and senior managers of ambulance trusts, senior leaders from policy and profes-sional bodies and international experts who lead, influence or manage the ambu-lance services thus informing the policy and guiding the practice. Given the scope of this volume, the chosen themes and topics reflect some of the key management challenges currently being witnessed by the ambulance services meriting further scholarly research and reflection.

This volume serves as a timely and comprehensive reference for academics, pro-fessionals and practitioners involved in the analysis, evaluation and reflection of the challenges faced by a modern ambulance service. It also provides students and social scientists with a critical understanding needed to build a scientific basis for interventions and addressing some of the issues raised and deliberated in this book. We hope that *Ambulance Services: Leadership and Management Perspectives* be-comes a credible resource for factual, critical and comprehensive information on the management perspectives of the twenty-first century pre-hospital care.

September 2015
Paresh Wankhade
Kevin Mackway-Jones

Acknowledgements

There are a number of people to whom we would like to express our sincere gratitude for this ambitious project. First, we would like to thank our authors who are well-regarded for the expertise in their respective fields. They range from senior academics, chief executives, senior managers, professional experts and independent practitioners. To bring them all together is a key highlight of this volume and to this end this is a book by the people who lead and manage the ambulance services and their opinions are important in informing the policy and guiding the practice. Second, to the team at Springer, in particular, we are grateful to Janice Stern and Christina Tuballes. Third, to Prof. George Talbot and Prof. James O'Kane at the Edge Hill University for supporting the project. And lastly to our families for allowing us, at different periods, to write this book.

Paresh Wankhade
Kevin Mackway-Jones

Contents

Part I   Context and Background

**1   Introduction: Understanding the Management of
    Ambulance Services**..   3
    Paresh Wankhade and Kevin Mackway-Jones

2   Historical Perspectives in the Ambulance Service................................   17
    Alexander Pollock

Part II   Providing Emergency Care

3   A Strategy for Managing Quality in Ambulance Services....................   31
    Mary Peters, Steve Barnard, Michael Dorrian and
    Kevin Mackway-Jones

4   Management of Emergency Demand...   43
    Bob Williams

5   Ethical Commissioning of Emergency Ambulance Services................   51
    Mark Docherty

Part III   Context of Emergency Care

**6   Organisational and Professional Cultures:
    An Ambulance Perspective**...   65
    Paresh Wankhade, James Radcliffe and Geoffrey Heath

**7   Leadership and System Thinking in the Modern
    Ambulance Service**..   81
    Andy Newton and Graham Harris

8 Ambulance Service Modernisation 95
   Robert Till and Anthony Marsh

9 Interoperability and Multiagency Cooperation 107
   John Stephenson

10 Responding to Diversity and Delivering Equality in
    Prehospital Care: Statutory Responsibilities, Best Practice
    and Recommendations 119
    Viet-Hai Phung, Karen Windle and A. Niroshan Siriwardena

11 Dealing with the Austerity Challenge 135
    Robert Till and Anthony Marsh

Part IV   Looking to the Future

12 The Ambulance Service of the Future 149
    Mark Docherty, Andrew Carson and Matthew Ward

13 Future Perspectives for the UK Ambulance Services:
    Evolution Rather than Revolution 157
    Kevin Mackway-Jones and Paresh Wankhade

14 International Perspectives: Australian
    Ambulance Services in 2020 163
    Paul M Middleton

15 International Perspectives: South African
    Ambulance Services in 2020 175
    Craig Vincent-Lambert

16 International Perspectives: Finnish Ambulance Services in 2020 185
    Juha Jormakka and Simo Saikko

Index 191

About the editors

Prof. Paresh Wankhade is a Professor of Leadership and Management at the Edge Hill University Business School. He has done his PhD in ambulance performance & culture change management from the University of Liverpool, UK. He is the founder editor of the *International Journal of Emergency Services* (an Emerald group Publication) and is recognised as an expert in the field of emergency management. He has chaired special tracks on leadership and management of emergency services at major international conferences including the annual European Academy of Management (EURAM) Conference, British Academy of Management Conference and Public Administration Committee (PAC) Conference. His research and publications focus on analyses of strategic leadership, organisational culture, organisational change and interoperability within the emergency services. His publications have contributed to inform debates around interoperability of public services and challenges faced by individual organisations. His latest book on *Social Capital, Sociability and Community Development* explores these issues including the state of the pre-hospital care in eight selected case study countries (UK, USA, China, India, Bangladesh, Japan, Netherlands and South Africa) around the world.

Prof. Kevin Mackway-Jones was appointed as a consultant at the Manchester Royal Infirmary in 1993 and became a professor in the year 2001. He has published widely on the practice and theory of emergency medicine, both books (*Advanced Paediatric Life Support, Major Incident Medical Management and Support, Emergency Triage* amongst others) and academic papers. His main research interests are diagnostic strategies, psychosocial care and major incident management. Apart from consulting at the Manchester Royal Infirmary and the Royal Manchester Children's Hospital he is also an executive medical director at the North West Ambulance Service, civilian consultant advisor to the British Army and head of the North Western School of Emergency Medicine. He is the webmaster for www.bestbets. org and the St Emlyn's Virtual Hospital through which he runs masters' degree in emergency medicine. He was an editor in chief of the *Emergency Medicine Journal* from 2005–2013.

Contributors

Steve Barnard North West Ambulance Service NHS Trust, Bolton, UK

Andrew Carson West Midlands Ambulance Service NHS Foundation Trust, Dudley, West Midlands, UK

Mark Docherty West Midlands Ambulance Service NHS Foundation Trust, Dudley, West Midlands, UK

Michael Dorrian North West Ambulance Service NHS Trust, Bolton, UK

Graham Harris College of Paramedics, Bridgwater, UK

Geoffrey Heath Keele Management School, Keele University, Keele, Staffordshire, UK

Juha Jormakka Department of Paramedic Nursing, Saimaa University of Applied Sciences, Lappeenranta, Skinnarillankatu 36, Finland

Kevin Mackway-Jones North West Ambulance Service NHS Trust, Bolton, UK

Anthony Marsh West Midlands Ambulance Service NHS FT, Brierley Hill, West Midlands, UK

Paul M Middleton Discipline of Emergency Medicine, University of Sydney/DREAM Collaboration, Sydney, NSW, Australia

Andy Newton South East Coast Ambulance Service, Banstead, Surrey, UK

Mary Peters North West Ambulance Service NHS Trust, Bolton, UK

Viet-Hai Phung Community and Health Research Unit, School of Health and Social Care, University of Lincoln, Lincoln, Lincolnshire, UK

Alexander Pollock Centre for the Study of the History of Medicine, Lilybank House, Bute Gardens, Glasgow G12 8RT, UK

James Radcliffe Faculty of Health Sciences, Staffordshire University, Stafford, UK

Simo Saikko Department of Paramedic Nursing, Saimaa University of Applied Sciences, Lappeenranta, Skinnarillankatu 36, Finland

A. Niroshan Siriwardena Community and Health Research Unit, School of Health and Social Care, University of Lincoln, Lincoln, Lincolnshire, UK

John Stephenson National Ambulance Resilience Unit (NARU), Police National CBRN Centre, Ryton on Dunsmore, Coventry, UK

Robert Till West Midlands Ambulance Service NHS FT, Brierley Hill, West Midlands, UK

Craig Vincent-Lambert Department of Emergency Medical Care, University of Johannesburg, Doornfontein, Johannesburg, South Africa

Paresh Wankhade Edge Hill Business School, Edge Hill University, Ormskirk, UK

Matthew Ward West Midlands Ambulance Service NHS Foundation Trust, Dudley, West Midlands, UK

Bob Williams North West Ambulance Service NHS Trust, Bolton, UK

Karen Windle Community and Health Research Unit, School of Health and Social Care, University of Lincoln, Lincoln, Lincolnshire, UK

Part I
Context and Background

Chapter 1
Introduction: Understanding the Management of Ambulance Services

Paresh Wankhade and Kevin Mackway-Jones

Context and Background

The origins of the ambulance service as a public service can be traced back to the late nineteenth and early twentieth centuries with the development of a horse-drawn service that was set up in Liverpool in 1883; the city of London Ambulance Service in 1906; and the introduction of the 999 service in 1937 (Ambulance Service Association 2000). When the National Health Service (NHS) was created in 1948, the ambulance service was a function given to the local authorities. Unlike the police and fire services, there was no accompanying legislation to provide structures and operational arrangements for the new ambulance services that were classified as 'essential' rather than 'emergency' services (IBID, p. 7). With a further absence of any infrastructure for leadership or training, individual services found their own ways of operating. Uniforms and rank structures emulated the established emergency services and a basic first aid certificate was all that was required to work in the services.

Since becoming a part of the wider NHS in 1974, ambulance services have made huge progress to develop from a simple transport service into a pre-hospital healthcare service. During the 1990s, ambulance services became NHS trusts. Prior to reorganisation in 2006, there were 31 ambulance trusts in England. Reorganisation created 11 trusts organised around government offices of the region boundaries

P. Wankhade (✉)
Edge Hill Business School, Edge Hill University, Room B204, L39 4QP Ormskirk, UK
e-mail: Paresh.Wankhade@edgehill.ac.uk

K. Mackway-Jones
North West Ambulance Service NHS Trust,
Ladybridge Hall, Chorley New Road, Heaton, BL1 5DD Bolton, UK
e-mail: kevin.Mackway-Jones@nwas.nhs.uk

© Springer International Publishing Switzerland 2015
P. Wankhade, K. Mackway-Jones (eds.), *Ambulance Services,*
DOI 10.1007/978-3-319-18642-9_1

(DH 2005, p. 10). All of these trusts provide both emergency and non-emergency services. Emergency transport is provided by individual ambulance trusts in response to 999 calls and urgent requests from general practitioners and clinicians including inter-hospital transfers using an emergency vehicle. The patient transport service (PTS) provides pre-booked carriage of patients to hospital, for example, to outpatient appointments and to daycare centres.

The ambulance service is the first point of access for a wide variety of health problems and is a gateway to the NHS in England. The significant gaps in the healthcare literature; especially in relation to paramedic care is characterised by the fact that most documented research revolves around specific episodes of medical care in hospitals or other permanent healthcare facilities (Linwood et al. 2007). The nature of the patient care in the ambulance services is more immediate and delivered under trying, and often unstable conditions. Patient care and research into how to improve the service in such circumstances, necessitates a different but complementary approach to that of other healthcare organisations (Tippett et al. 2003; Woods et al. 2002). The pre-hospital and emergency medical systems (EMS) research lags behind other health disciplines and medical specialties, and there is a need to increase the profile, and volume, of pre-hospital research especially from a public policy and management perspective (Andrews and Wankhade 2014; Wankhade 2011a, 2012; Heath and Radcliffe 2007, 2010; Bevan and Hood 2006).

The management interest in the working of the ambulance services is surprisingly a recent phenomenon given the fact the saving and caring for the wounded or the sick and injured dates back to ancient times (Pollock 2013; Caple 2004; Wankhade and Murphy 2012). Unlike other sectors (acute trusts, primary care trusts and specialist trusts) within the NHS, management explorations about the ambulance services is a comparatively less researched phenomenon in the growing discourse around emergency management (Wankhade 2011a, 2012; McCann et al. 2013; Wankhade and Brinkman 2014; Heath and Radcliffe 2007). Historically, the ambulance services have been viewed primarily as a call-handling and transportation service, incorporating some aspects of patient care. Increasingly, their wider role as an outlet to other NHS services and in ensuring that patients can access the facilities closer to their home is being recognised (NAO 2011).

In keeping with this enhanced role of the ambulance services, the first national ambulance review (DH 2005, p. 14) provided a blue print for ambulance modernisation and future roadmap. The vision of the government was identified to improve the speed and quality of call handling to ensure consistent telephone services for patients who need urgent care. To achieve this vision, developing leadership capability—clinical and managerial—was identified to be reinforced and developed along with education, learning and development for all staff to meet the professional standards expected of them. The period from 2006 to 2010, witnessed contradictory policy objectives. Ambulance services were expected to implement the vision set out in the national review through an enhanced role of the emergency care practitioners (ECPs) but grapple simultaneously with the upheavals and challenges of reorganisation and still show performance. The reliance on the response time targets for measuring ambulance performance was also the subject of focus of some of the earlier published management research for promoting gaming and manipulating results (Bevan and Hamblin 2009; Bevan and Hood 2006). In the quest for standardisation, the government introduced the new 8-min standard *Call to Connect* which further made the meeting of the target difficult (Woollard et al. 2010; Wankhade 2011b). Thus, the performance management regime for ambulance services exemplified the potential of performance measures to promote dysfunctional behaviour as it fell into many of the pitfalls identified in the literature (Heath and Wankhade 2014; De Bruijn 2002; Radcliffe and Heath 2009).

Developing general practice (GP) commissioning was the centrepiece of the reforms announced by the coalition government in 2010. This was accompanied by the introduction of a range of clinical performance indicators for ambulance services which came into effect in April, 2011. The urgent and life-threatening targets are still in practice but a set of new 11 indicators have been introduced (see Cooke 2011 for a fuller discussion; DH 2010a). Additionally, since April 2010, ambulance services like the other NHS organisations also annually publish the *Quality Accounts* intending to promote the overall quality of the service provided and benchmarking of performance (DH 2010b, 2012). Thus, the ambulance trusts are currently focussed to play an enhanced role on one hand in upskilling the staff and paramedic crews and their professionalisation (see NHS England 2013; McCann et al. 2013) and on the other hand, to confront organisational change by exploring alternate models of patient treatment at the scene or at home eliminating the need for hospital admissions (Lovegrove and Davis 2013; NHS Confederation 2014). However, ambulance trusts are still battling some of the legacy issues especially around a *'uniform culture'* which does not always sit comfortably with the core NHS values. Few of the issues surrounding occupational cultures and group identities coupled with the reliance on response time targets and options to 'treat and refer' (O'Cathain et al. 2014) on the backdrop of a growing demand of emergency 999 calls is having its own unintended consequences (Smith 1995; Wankhade and Brinkman 2014; Wankhade 2011a). This volume will explore key management issues being experienced by the ambulance trusts in the UK in dealing with some of these challenges.

Realty and Perception

In 2009–2010, the cost of ambulance services was £1.9 billion, of which £1.5 billion was for urgent and emergency services (NAO 2011). However with an annual budget of more than a £2 billion in 2013–2014 (NHS England 2013) and an overexpanding portfolio of services offered by the emergency ambulance services, their contribution is quite significant (Her Majesty's HM Treasury, 2010). The fundamental principle of providing a comprehensive service to the patients, with the access based upon clinical needs and not their ability to pay for the services offered by the NHS has been seriously tested by the urgent and emergency care in England (NHS England 2013). Several factors have contributed to the ongoing challenges faced by urgent and emergency care networks. These include, among other things,

Table 1.1 Growing demand of emergency calls in England. (Adapted from Health and Social Care Information Centre 2013)

Year	Number of calls in thousands
2004–2005	5623.8
2005–2006	5960.1
2006–2007	6333.4
2007–2008	7225.5
2008–2009	7447.2
2009–2010	7867.9
2010–2011	8077.5
2011–2012	9493.0
2012–2013	9081.0

an annual rise in the demand of emergency 999 calls (see Table 1.1) which have grown on an average annual rate of 4–6%. During 2012–2013, there was an increase of 6–9% over the previous year for the total number of emergency calls received (see Table 1.2).

Furthermore, the alternate delivery protocols and delivery are focus of current management and academic attention (AACE 2014; Siriwardena et al. 2010; Snookes et al. 2009). There have been relatively few detailed explorations of the dynamics of the ambulance services in terms of their management; the relationship between different groups of employees; and the impact of organisational culture in improving the quality of service delivery (Wankhade 2012). This volume attempts to address this gap.

Table 1.2 Key facts about the ambulance services in England in 2012–2013. (Source: Health and Social Care Information Centre 2013)

1. The total number of emergency calls was 9.08 million, a 587,972 (6.9%) increase over last year when there were 8.49 million. Of these, 2.95 million (32.5%) were category A (immediately life threatening). Of all calls, 6.98 million (76.9%) resulted in an emergency response arriving at the scene of the incident, a 268,472 (4.0%) increase over last year when there were 6.71 million

2. The percentage of category A (immediately life threatening) incidents that resulted in an emergency response arriving at the scene of the incident within 8 min in 2012–2013 was:
(a) 75.5% (April–May)
(b) 74.0% (Red 1, June–March)
(c) 75.6% (Red 2, June–March)

3. Of the 12 NHS organisations providing ambulance services, the following number met or exceeded the 75% standard for 8-min response times.
(a) 9 met or exceeded 75% (April–May)
(b) 7 met or exceeded 75% (Red 1, June–April)
(c) 11 met or exceeded 75% (Red 2, June–April)

4. The percentage of category A incidents that resulted in an ambulance vehicle capable of transporting the patient arriving at the scene within 19 min was 96.0% (AQI data). Last year this was 96.8% (KA34); however, these data are not directly comparable due to different clock start times

NHS National Health Service

Aims and Plan of This Book

This is the second book in a three volume series on the management of the three blue light emergency services (ambulance, police and the fire and rescue services). This volume aims to provide a broader management understanding of the ambulance services which would be of equal interest to students, academics, practitioners and professionals without compromising the rigour and scholarship of the content. We have invited experts in their particular fields to address the chosen themes, in both the theory and practice of the functioning of the ambulance services in the UK. The key thinking in this volume is to provide a broad understanding of the major management issues relevant to the operation of the ambulance services in the UK along with an international perspective. Admittedly, it is a difficult endeavour to cover all the possible management themes in a single volume such as this but we are confident that the chosen themes will give a rounded understanding and insights into the management of the ambulance services. The current available texts do not provide such an expert and balanced view on the management of the ambulance services.

This volume provides a mature understanding of an emergency service, which hitherto, is neglected in the management research. Thus, one of the aims of this volume is to invite a new generation of management scholars to explore the study of the ambulance services. This volume will also appeal to a range of students (both undergraduate and postgraduate) studying organisational theory as well as social sciences, sociology, economics and politics, public health, and emergency and disaster management. The book offers critical insights into the theory and practise of strategic and operational management of ambulance services and the related professional and policy aspects. For a large number of staff working in the emergency care settings, the growing calls for professionalisation of the service (through closer links with Higher Education Institutions (HEIs)) and the recognition to reflect on their own personal development, this volume seeks to provide an authoritative source on the management of the ambulance services addressing the knowledge gaps. To a growing audience of independent practitioners and consultants, this volume will appeal in equal measure.

More attention is being paid now to the management research on ambulance services given the policy and practice implications of the challenges to the urgent and emergency care settings. Several factors have contributed towards the need for a better understanding of the role and contribution of the ambulance services in the wider health economy. The pressures on hospital accident and emergency (A&Es) units and the resulting delays for the ambulance crews have been well rehearsed. The limited options for out-of-hours care and a growing ageing population will add more pressures on the use of the ambulance services. The Mid Staffordshire Hospital Inquiry (Francis 2013) and the Keogh Review (NHS England 2013) both highlighted a cultural transformation of the hospital and emergency/urgent care services in England. This requires a better understanding of these issues making this project particularly timely. The chosen themes in this volume will help to outline the social, cultural and political context in which the ambulance services is to be understood. This volume covers issues of theory, policy and practice and raises questions, some of which are inherently controversial. Each of the chapters seeks to engage with the current debates about the direction of travel. The contributors also examine the latest development in their chosen field of enquiry. This volume thus aims to set out the management understanding of the ambulance services as a significant subdiscipline of emergency management and also provide a basis of learning and teaching in this field.

One of the other aims of this volume is to bring together top-quality scholarship using experts—academics, practitioners and professionals in the field to each of the chosen topics. Admittedly, this was an ambitious task and we have been really fortunate to have an assembly of authors who are well regarded for the expertise in their fields. They range from senior academics, chief executives and senior managers from the NHS and independent practitioners. To bring them all together is a key highlight of this volume and to this end this is a book by the people who lead and manage the ambulance services, and their opinions are important in informing the policy and guiding the practice. The contributors have written from different perspectives of critical academics to chief executives and policy experts and there is much to be gained from reading chapters in conjunction with each other, contrasting different perspectives and approaches (Newburn 2003, p. 7). We are immensely grateful to them for their untiring work that has gone to produce this volume and feel confident that it will do justice to the complexities of the chosen themes. All the chapters have been completed in 2014–2015 and hence draw upon the latest evidence and research base available on the chosen topic. The chapters are based in the practical experiences of the authors and are written in a way that is accessible and suitable for a range of audiences.

In dealing with these issues, the volume is divided into four parts. Part 1 provides the context and background to this volume. In this chapter, we have examined the state of the management research on the ambulance services and have stated the aims of this volume. In Chap. 2, Alex Pollock provides an historical context to the origins of the ambulance services. He argues that for most of human history, the care of the wounded in war or the sick and injured in the community was not of great concern to generals or those in civil authority. Exceptions existed but these did not lead to a general movement towards the provision of ambulance services on the battlefield or the street. Then in 1792, a surgeon in the Napoleonic army designed the first threefold system of good military ambulance practice, treating the wounded in situ, speedily transporting them from the place of conflict and providing a safe facility for aftercare. In 1866, a doctor in New York organised the first civil ambulance service which was summoned by telegraph, thereby completing the four features upon which modern ambulance services are based: dedicated teams, standby vehicles, reception hospitals and electronic communication. After slow and uncertain beginnings, ambulances began to save increasing numbers of lives using ingenuity and technological innovation since becoming part of the NHS in 1974.

Part 2 of this volume deals with the working of the ambulance services in providing emergency care to patients. Three key themes are examined. In Chap. 3, problematic issue of managing 'quality' and 'risk' is tackled by Mary Peters, Steve

Barnard, Michael Doorian and Kevin-Mackway-Jones. They argue that while the practice of risk management and corporate governance relates to all aspects of an organisation's business and activities, the current focus within the health service is primarily around improving quality by putting the patient first and protecting them from harm and developing a culture of transparency and openness (for instance, the NHS Outcome Framework). The measurement of quality within ambulance services has also been traditionally limited to operational activities and presents significant challenges due to the unique environment they operate within, in comparison to other types of healthcare providers. Ambulance services across England use the Clinical Performance Indicator Care Bundle to measure and monitor the quality of care given to patients. Reviewing the current state of development of ambulance quality indicators, the authors conclude that the care received by patients in the pre-hospital arena could be measured and monitored using the Clinical Leadership Education Accountability and Responsibility (CLEAR) framework.

In Chap. 4, Bob Williams examines the core but increasingly difficult issue of managing the demand for ambulance calls. He argues whether it is time to consider remodelling the English ambulance services in order to meet the competing requirements of public expectation and rising emergency demand against the backdrop of a reducing financial position and significant changes to the healthcare system and the incident mix now being attended. He further argues that the underlying increase in demand for ambulance services is universal with a number of similar themes emanating from socio-demographic changes of ageing and multiple illnesses combined with an urbanisation and fragmentation of communities. This has resulted in ambulance services starting to struggle with meeting the exacting response standards expected for potential emergencies irrespective of demographics or geography, while also providing an acceptable service in the eyes of the public to less urgent but nonetheless individually concerning health concerns.

In Chap. 5, the issue of commissioning of the ambulance service is investigated by Mark Docherty. Urgent and Emergency ambulance services are a critical part of the pre-hospital infrastructure and are held in high regard with service users and the public. These services are working in a challenging climate where decisions on priority setting have to be made within an ethically acceptable framework. Commissioners of ambulance services need to ensure that services that are in place are effective (do good) and that decisions on priority setting are fair. For ambulance services the principles of ethical commissioning will not always reach a conclusion on priority setting, and a triangulated approach that also includes clinicians, service users and the public in decision making will ensure that a decision is fair, and the process for decision making is open and transparent resulting in a more ethically robust decision that has greater legitimacy.

Part 3 of the volume explores the context of emergency care through six key themes. The issue of ambulance and professional culture(s) is examined first by Paresh Wankhade, James Radcliffe and Geoffrey Heath in Chap. 6. This chapter concerns the place of culture in ambulance services. There are issues around organisational cultures and subcultures, and the ways these are cross-cut by professional cultures. The concept of organisational culture looms large in recent literature on organisational change, but this is problematic. It is difficult to define culture adequately and the ways in which it affects behaviour are obscure. In the case of ambulance services, for instance, does it make sense to refer to a single culture within, let alone across, organisations? Similarly, can cultures be transformed as easily as sometimes suggested? Nevertheless, governments increasingly seek to move the focus in the NHS from changing structures and systems towards changing cultures. This raises a number of interesting questions. What happens when attempts to change organisational cultures encounter professional cultures, which support power and status based on professional standing? What are the implications of attempting to professionalise other NHS occupational groups (such as ambulance personnel)? This is particularly relevant given the changing role of ambulance paramedics, which is an international phenomenon. ECPs now have the skills to carry out a wider range of activities at the scene of incidents, and there is increasing evidence of effectiveness. However, this requires services to become 'learning organisations' providing continuous training and development, but it is still questionable whether the cultures and subcultures of ambulance services support what may be seen as an imposed initiative. Thus, there are examples of variations in training and of ECPs not being utilised fully. In analysing these issues, Schein's identification of pluralistic dimensions of culture has been used. The authors conclude that ambulance organisations have multiple cultures, some of which counter change. This complexity adds to the difficulties of delivering effective reforms.

Chapter 7 deals with the issue of leadership development in the ambulance service. Andy Newton and Graham Harris make a strong case for leadership and system thinking in the modern ambulance service arguing that ambulance services remain locked in an eighteenth century mind-set that reinforces a traditional emergency care and transport focused mode of operation, which is insufficiently attuned to the changing and more heterogeneous actualities of demand of the modern world. An effective response to current rising pressures will require clear doctrine and revised concept of operation that is far more reflective of contemporary epidemiological realities and the changing role of the Ambulance Service and the Paramedics. They conclude that effecting the necessary organisational and professional changes will require both a high order of leadership and the recognition that there is a fundamental relationship between leadership and the design of the system in which leadership is being practiced.

In Chap. 8, Robert Till and Anthony Marsh explore the issue of ambulance service modernisation by setting the scene regarding the challenges the ambulance services are currently facing. The authors then goes on to discuss the ways in which the ambulance service have responded to these challenges and what methods have been adopted to improve patient care while also creating efficiencies.

Our next expert John Stephenson deals with the subject of interoperability and multi-agency cooperation in Chap. 9. He discusses how the UK emergency services have worked together for many years, but repeatedly at major incidents, they have settled back into silo working, and how a major programme to train commanders to work differently and understand each other's issues only started in 2013. It is further argued that the issue of interoperability is very dependent on the organisational structure within each country. In the UK the police, fire and ambulance services are very separate and the armed forces are rarely called upon to support homeland activities except when a specific issue requiring their skills or manpower is identified. Outside the UK, it is common for ambulance services to be provided to some extent within the fire services, this is largely a small cadre of staff that respond to the significant traumatic incidents and very sick collapsed patients, and the broader ambulance work is often provided by private organisations rather than as an emergency service.

The subject matter of responding to diversity and delivering equality in prehospital care is next examined in Chap. 10 by our experts Viet-Hai Phung, Karen Windle and Niroshan Siriwardena. Population and workforce diversity in the NHS together with legislation and national guidance has led to equality becoming an increasingly important issue for patients, service users and staff. Ambulance services, as public sector organisations, are bound by the Equality Act 2010, and as NHS organisations are actively encouraged to implement the Equality Delivery System (EDS) and its successor EDS2, providing the local strategic context to understand and address system inequalities. This chapter examines current challenges for ambulance services in relation to equality and why this matters. It goes on to explore how services are responding to diversity, how they should embed this through engagement with both patients and staff, and how they should understand the effects of these activities through more effective data monitoring.

In Chap. 11, the problem of dealing with the massive challenges of cuts in the NHS budgets is considered by Robert Till and Anthony Marsh. They examine the challenges faced by the NHS ambulance trusts in England in doing 'more for less' and coping with the austerity. This chapter describes the difficult financial position the NHS faces and how this directly affects the ambulance services. It discusses the changing demographics and attitude of the UK and the impact of these on the ambulance services. The authors go onto discuss the innovative ideas and changes ambulance services have had to make to meet the ever-increasing demand placed upon them. Finally, the question is raised regarding the possible need for a change in commissioning of the ambulance services.

Part 4 of this volume presents different perspectives on the future of the ambulance services both in the UK and abroad. In Chap. 12, the first contribution by Mark Docherty, Andrew Carson and Matthew Ward highlights the new agenda for development of clinical skills and a new perspective on the future of ambulance services. The authors discuss how ambulance services historically and up until recently have been predominantly a transport service for sick and injured people, and the development of ambulance services for delivery of clinical services has happened sporadically and slowly during this period. They contend that pre-hospital urgent and emergency care is changing rapidly, and the twenty-first century will see the need for ambulance services to change at an exponential rate. They conclude that demand on ambulance services caused by the growing elderly population and expectations of the younger generation provide a great opportunity and a challenge for the current service to develop into modern providers of mobile health services that have a relevance in a twenty-first century healthcare system.

Kevin Mackway-Jones and Paresh Wankhade in their piece argue the case for a sensible understanding of the challenges being faced by ambulance trusts in England in Chap. 13. They contend that the future of ambulance services raises important issues about the nature of prehospital care and the changing societal and cultural context in the UK. They highlight two core functions of the ambulance services—a means of supported transport of patients in the community and a responsive and professional outreaching emergency diagnosis and management service. Their view is that while these functions will still be integral in the future pre-hospital care models, what is likely to change is the means of delivery and the professionals that deliver the service. They conclude their arguments by making a case for an evolutionary change than rather than change by revolution which essentially centres on the 3Ss- structure, skills and science.

In Chaps. 14-16, we present three contributions addressing international perspectives for the ambulance services. Our first expert Paul Middleton reviews the provision of ambulance service delivery in Australia in Chap. 14. He argues that ambulance services by 2020 should be having the ability to analyse and measure the quality of systems and processes in relation to patient outcomes. Adherence to the current system of targets for response times based on medians from other jurisdictions remote in geography, time and design will need to be replaced with carefully analysed linked data using sophisticated statistical techniques, including regression and survival analyses as well as comprehensive health economic evaluations, to allow patient outcomes to be utilised to determine the effectiveness of ambulance practice. Based upon his analysis, the author concludes that only when the ambulance systems are joined to health services, Australian ambulance services truly will have come into the twenty-first century.

In Chap. 15, our second expert Craig Lambert analyses the pre-hospital care and ambulance service delivery in South Africa where the training and scope of practice of ambulance personal differs vastly between different regions within the country. Certain EMSs offer a doctor-based system with medical doctors responding on emergency vehicles to calls while at the other end of the spectrum are EMSs that operate with ambulance crews that have as little as 3–4 weeks of basic training. The chapter details how emergency care profession has developed away from a doctor-driven technician system towards a more autonomous profession and by implication, the responsibility for clinical decision making, interrogation, critique and development of pre-hospital medical protocol and direction is now largely driven by the paramedics. The author concludes that the extent to which this fledgling autonomous profession is capable of properly fulfilling these important functions is frequently debated.

Our final international contributors Juha Jormakka and Simo Saikko share an expert perspective on the Finnish ambulance services in Chap. 16. They begin with a short history of ambulance service in Finland and the development of educational standards in paramedic practice within the context of Europe including the continuing education and professional development agenda. They provide an insight about the quality factors and risk management issues while evaluating the effectiveness of treating ring people at home sketching the future direction of travel.

Limitations of the Current Project

There were a few difficult decisions we had to take as editors of this volume; the biggest one was to decide what to include in the volume of this and what was to be excluded. We are also conscious about the possible disagreements about the final contents of the volume and what else could or should have been covered. Furthermore, even the scope of some of the chapters could have been more detailed and capable of being examined in a greater detail. The chosen themes do not claim to cover the whole gamut of issues which could be applied to the management of ambulance services. Nonetheless, they provide a fair representation of topics that concern us in our scholarly research and teaching. We firmly believe that they represent opportunities for both teaching and practice to reflect on these issues. We also seriously deliberated upon the choice of the authors and their backgrounds. In the end, we were convinced that a choice reflecting a balance between academic experts and senior practitioners would allow bringing greater criticality and reflection to understand the complexity of the chosen themes. Rather than having rigid guidelines over chapter style and structures, we saw greater relevance in a 'light touch', free-flowing style of each of the chapters in presenting contrasting perspectives from academics and practitioners. We are of the opinion that this approach worked better in a work like this though it will be for our readers to judge whether we were correct in our methodology. Similarly, we could have paid more attention to the developments in the urgent and emergency care outside England including some comparative outlooks though there remains a strong comparative element from Australia, South Africa and Finland.

Future Research Agenda

Ambulance services often provide the first point of contact in the global healthcare systems. But the context in which they currently operate within the urgent and emergency care settings is increasingly becoming fragmented, complex and politically contested. The pressures of funding, training and cultural transformation are now felt globally. The need to learn and adapt from suitable models of ambulance service delivery across the globe have never been greater. We sincerely hope that this volume will trigger greater academic and organisational interest in the understanding of one of the most important of public services. We aim to further work on a comparative element outside the UK and invite interested colleagues and partners to join the quest of the management understanding of a service we love so dearly.

Bibliography

Association of Ambulance Chief Executives (AACE). (2014). *Annual Report-2013–2014.* London: AACE.

Ambulance Service Association. (2000). The future of ambulance services in the United Kingdom: A strategic review of options for the future of ambulance services. *Medical care Research Unit: The University of Sheffield* (on behalf of the Ambulance Service Association).

Andrews, R., & Wankhade, P. (2014). Regional variations in emergency service performance: Does social capital matter? *Regional Studies.* doi:10.1080/00343404.2014.891009.

Bevan, G., & Hamblin, R. (2009). Hitting and missing targets by ambulance services for emergency calls: Effects of different systems of performance measurement within the UK. *Journal of the Royal Statistical Society, 172*(1), 161–190.

Bevan, G., & Hood, C. (2006). What's measured is what matters: Targets and gaming in the English Public Health Care System. *Public Administration, 84*(3), 517–538.

Caple, L. (2004). *From ambulances to almonds.* Victoria: Trafford.

Cooke, M. (2011). An introduction to the new ambulance clinical quality indicators. *Ambulance Today, 7*(5), 35–39.

De Bruijn, H. (2002). *Managing performance in the public sector.* London: Routledge.

Department of Health (DH). (2005). *Taking healthcare to the patients: Transforming NHS ambulance services.* London: Department of Health.

Department of Health (DH). (2010a). Reforming urgent and emergency care performance management. www.dh.gov.uk/en/Healthcare/Urgentandemergencycare/DH_121239. Accessed 15 June 2014.

Department of Health (DH) (2010b). Quality Accounts toolkit 2010/11. www.dh.gov.uk/publications-. Accessed 18 June 2014.

Department of Health (DH) (2012). Quality Account audit and future reporting changes advised. www.dh.gov.uk/health/2012/02/quality-account-reporting/. Accessed 6 July 2014.

Francis, R. (2013). *Mid Staffordshire NHS Foundation Trust Public Inquiry.* Final Report. London: The Stationery Office.

Heath, G., & Radcliffe, J. (2007). Performance measurement and the English ambulance service. *Public Money & Management, 27*(3), 223–227.

Heath, G., & Radcliffe, J. (2010). Exploring the utility of current performance measures for changing roles and practices of ambulance paramedics. *Public Money & Management, 30*(3), 151–158.

Heath, G., & Wankhade, P. (2014). A balanced judgement? Performance indicators, quality and the english ambulance service; some issues, developments and a research agenda. *The Journal of Finance and Management in Public Services, 13*(1) (Early cite).

Her Majesty's Treasury (2010) *Spending Review,* 2010, CM 7942. The Stationery Office: London.

Health and Social Care Information Centre. (2013). Ambulance services, England—2012–13 and Emergency calls (1) by ambulance service, 2004–05 to 2012–13. http://www.hscic.gov.uk/searchcatalogue?productid 11839&q=title%3a%22Ambulance+Services%2c+England%22&sort=Relevance&size=10&page=1#top. Accessed 10 July 2014.

Linwood, R., Day, G., Fitzgerald, G., & Oldenburg, B. (2007). Quality Improvement and paramedic care- What does the literature reveal for pre-hospital emergency care in Australia? *International Journal of Health Care Quality Assurance, 20*(5), 405–415.

Lovegrove, M., & Davis, J., (2013). *Maximising paramedics' contribution to the delivery of high quality and cost effective patient care.* High Wycombe: Buckinghamshire New University.

McCann, J., Granter, E., Hyde, P., & Hassard, J. (2013). Still blue-collar after all these years? An ethnography of the professionalization of emergency ambulance work. *Journal of Management Studies, 50*(5), 750–776.

National Audit Office (NAO). (2011). *Transforming NHS ambulance services. Report by the Comptroller and Auditor General HC 1086.* London: The Stationery Office.

Newburn, T. (2003). *Handbook of policing.* Cullompton: Willan.

NHS Confederation. (2014). *Ripping off the sticking plaster: Whole-systems solutions for urgent and emergency care*. London: NHS Confederation.

NHS England. (2013). *Transforming urgent and emergency care in England: Urgent and emergency care review, Phase 1 Report*. Leeds: NHS England.

O'Cathain, A., Knowles, E., Maheswaran, R., Pearson, T., Turner, J., & Hirst, E. (2014). A systemwide approach to explaining variation in potentially avoidable emergency admissions: National ecological study. *BMJ Quality and Safety, 23*(1), 47–55.

Pollock, A. C. (2013). Ambulance services in London and Great Britain from 1860 until today: A glimpse of history gleaned mainly from the pages of contemporary journals. *Emergency Medicine Journal, 30*(2), 218–222.

Radcliffe, J., & Heath, G. (2009). Ambulance calls and cancellations: Policy and implementation issues. *International Journal of Public Sector Management, 22*(5), 410–422.

Smith, P.C. (1995). On the unintended consequences of publishing performance data in the public sector. *International Journal of Public Administration, 18*(2/3), 277–310.

Snooks, H., Evans, A., Wells, B., Peconi, J., Thomas, M., Woollard, M., Guly, H., Jenkinson, E., Turner, J., & Hartley-Sharpe, C. (2009). What are the highest priorities for research in emergency prehospital care? *Emergency Medicine Journal, 26*(2), 549–550.

Siriwardena, A. N., Donohoe, R., & Stephenson, J. (2010). Supporting research and development in ambulance services: Research for better health care in prehospital settings. *Emergency Medicine Journal, 27*(4), 324–326.

Tippett, V., Clark, M., Woods, S., & FitzGerald, G. (2003). Towards a national research agenda for the ambulance and pre-hospital sector in Australia. *Journal of Emergency Primary Health Care, 1*(1/2), 1–8.

Wankhade, P. (2011a). Performance measurement and the UK emergency ambulance service: Unintended consequences of the ambulance response time targets. *International Journal of Public Sector Management, 24*(5), 384–402.

Wankhade, P. (2011b). Emergency services in austerity: Challenges, opportunities and future perspectives for the ambulance service in the UK. *Ambulance Today, 8*(5), 13–15.

Wankhade, P. (2012). Different cultures of management and their relationships with organizational performance: Evidence from the UK ambulance service. *Public Money & Management, 32*(5), 381–388.

Wankhade, P., & Brinkman, J. (2014). The negative consequences of culture change management: Evidence from a UK NHS ambulance service. *International Journal of Public Sector Management, 27*(1), 2–25.

Wankhade, P., & Murphy, P. (2012). Bridging the theory and practice gap in emergency services research: Case for a new journal. *International Journal of Emergency Services, 1*(1), 4–9.

Woods, S., Clark, M., & FitzGerald, G. (2002). *Queensland ambulance service: A case study in organisational reform*. Brisbane: Australian Centre for Pre-Hospital Care.

Woollard, M., O'Meara, P., & Munro, G. (2010). What price 90 s: Is "Call to Connect" a disservice to 999 callers? *Emergency Medicine Journal, 27*(10), 729–730.

Prof. Paresh Wankhade is a Professor of Leadership and Management at the Edge Hill University Business School. He has done his PhD in Ambulance Performance & Culture Change Management from the University of Liverpool, UK. He is the founder editor of the *International Journal of Emergency Services* (an Emerald group Publication) and is recognised as an expert in the field of emergency management. He has chaired special tracks on leadership and management of emergency services at major international conferences including the annual European Academy of Management (EURAM) Conference, British Academy of Management Conference and Public Administration Committee (PAC) Conference. His research and publications focus on analyses of strategic leadership, organisational culture, organisational change and interoperability within the emergency services. His publications have contributed to inform debates around interoperability of public services and challenges faced by individual organisations. His latest book on

Social Capital, Sociability and Community Development explores these issues including the state of the pre-hospital care in eight selected case study countries (UK, USA, China, India, Bangladesh, Japan, Netherlands and South Africa) around the world.

Prof. Kevin Mackway-Jones was appointed as a consultant at the Manchester Royal Infirmary in 1993 and became a professor in the year 2001. He has published widely on the practice and theory of Emergency Medicine, both books (*Advanced Paediatric Life Support, Major Incident Medical Management and Support, Emergency Triage* amongst others) and academic papers. His main research interests are diagnostic strategies, psychosocial care and major incident management. Apart from consulting at the Manchester Royal Infirmary and the Royal Manchester Children's Hospital, he is also an executive medical director at the North West Ambulance Service, civilian consultant advisor to the British Army and head of the North Western School of Emergency Medicine. He is the webmaster for www.bestbets.org and the St Emlyn's Virtual Hospital through which he runs an MSc in Emergency Medicine. He was an editor in chief of the *Emergency Medicine Journal* from 2005–2013.

Chapter 2
Historical Perspectives in the Ambulance Service

Alexander Pollock

Introduction

The *Concise Oxford English Dictionary* defines an ambulance as 'a vehicle equipped for taking sick or injured people to and from hospital'. Its nineteenth-century origins come from the French, 'hôpital ambulant', a mobile field hospital (Stevenson and Waite 2011, p. 41). In the history of the ambulance, almost any kind of transport has been employed to move the sick and injured, including stretchers, modified hand-carts, carriages and wagons drawn by oxen, horses, donkeys or mules, motorised vehicles, trains, ships and different types of aircraft. Non-emergency cases whose infirmity prevents their use of everyday transport may also use ambulances. The first military ambulance service provided injury stabilisation with ongoing necessary interventions en route, besides extraction from the location of the incident and conveyance to a place of care. These concepts were later developed at varying rates over the next 200 years in military and civilian contexts, although for most of the period ambulances were simply modes of patient transport with few refinements.

The Wounded in Battle

From the earliest times of human conflict, wounded soldiers were usually left on the battlefield, often for days, to die of thirst, cold or their wounds, being vulnerable to summary execution and looting by their enemies. Those who were recovered were transported by their compatriots to a place of care by whatever means was available

A. Pollock (✉)
Centre for the Study of the History of Medicine, Lilybank House,
Bute Gardens, Glasgow G12 8RT , UK
e-mail: pollock352@btinternet.com

© Springer International Publishing Switzerland 2015
P. Wankhade, K. Mackway-Jones (eds.), *Ambulance Services,*
DOI 10.1007/978-3-319-18642-9_2

to carry them. Potentially salvageable patients were lost because of long delays which caused the condition of survivors to deteriorate greatly. Philip II (382–336 BC), the father of Alexander the Great attached doctors and surgeons to each of his fighting units ('numeri', equivalent to a modern battalion of 350–400 men) and rewarded his stretcher bearers for bringing in men wounded in battle. Roman armies also gathered and cared for their wounded in battle. In the sixth century AD, the armies of the Byzantine Emperor Mauricius had squads of horsemen set aside with suitably modified saddles to take wounded men to medical tents prepared for their care (Bell 2009, pp. 3–10). In the eleventh century, crusaders provided wagons to carry their wounded and sick soldiers to tents specially erected for them to provide a place of treatment at the baggage train before being transported to hospitals in Jerusalem. Later, their carers were formed into nursing orders who continued to provide institutional care for the sick throughout Europe in the centuries which followed. Around 1476, Queen Isabella of Spain ordered the creation of specially constructed wagons for transporting wounded soldiers, and the concept was adopted by different armies throughout Europe (Bell 2009, p. 11).

By the mid-eighteenth century, most of Europe's armies had accompanying physicians and surgeons, as well as different forms of fixed and ambulant hospitals (Haller 2011, p. 11). However, none of them had ambulance services to remove the wounded from the field. Dominique-Jean Larrey, a French surgeon working in Napoleon's army in 1792, witnessed the fate of French soldiers at the battle of Limbourg, where the wounded lay for more than 24 h before attempts were made to recover them. To remedy this situation, Larrey devised a comprehensive ambulance service to avoid delays, with surgeons and attendants *(escouades volants)* treating casualties under fire before removing them on special carriages designed by him (Williams 1843, p. 225). They were called 'ambulance volontes', being based on a Napoleonic horse-drawn two-wheeled gun carriage which was taken onto the battlefield to evacuate the wounded to the safety of temporary tented hospitals for further treatment before removing them to conventional hospitals if necessary. Such temporary tented hospitals were also called 'ambulances' until the mid-nineteenth century after which time the term 'field hospital' was appearing and the word ambulance being applied to the means of transport. Larrey's transport system competed with Baron Percy's 'wurst wagon' which was a horse-drawn wagon packed with surgical instruments and dressings upon which surgeons and medical attendants were conveyed to the battlefield (Bell 2009, pp. 18–22). Larrey also designed four-wheeled wagons for transporting wounded on uneven terrain. His ambulance system of on-site treatment, evacuation and mobile field hospitals became a model for modern military ambulance services.

Wellington's army, in the 1808–1814 peninsular campaign against Napoleon, had no form of ambulance service whatsoever. When his soldiers were wounded, they were carried back to a dressing station, taking four men out of the fighting line. Twenty-four stretchers were provided initially for the campaign, but they were too heavy to carry, soldiers preferring improvised stretchers made of poles and blankets or just blankets, to evacuate the wounded from the field to be treated at dressing stations behind the lines, by regimental surgeons. Accounts of the circumstances under which they worked suggest that chaos was the order of the day and officers were preferentially treated before the ranks (Howard 2008, pp. 48–73). When James MacGrigor, Wellington's chief of the medical department was injured by a kick from a horse and could not keep up with the army, Wellington sent his personal carriage to pick him up, there being none other available (*The Lancet* 1900). Wellington objected to the use of any vehicle which could get in the way of his manoeuvres and was reluctant to provide dedicated wagons for casualties. However, after discovering that the army's own military wagons were almost unusable in the field, he allowed his surgeons to use them for transporting wounded after surgery. Locally hired ox-carts and wagons were also employed. At the end of this war, there were British soldiers in many hospitals all over the Iberian Peninsula where the fighting had taken place. None of the failures of care for British casualties led to public criticism in the UK, and it was 60 years after Waterloo that the British army formed a proper trained ambulance corps (Howard 2008, pp. 102–109).

The British army went to war in the Crimea in 1853 with 20 two-wheeled wagons and 20 four-wheeled wagons for transporting wounded from the battlefield to field hospitals, but, at times, they were not in the right place at the right time. The design of the ambulance wagons in use during the Crimean War was criticised in the medical correspondence of the time for being heavy and lumbering, and a proposal was made that it be redesigned to be lighter and more manoeuvrable (*British Medical Journal* 1858). At the start of the British army's campaign, advanced skirmishing parties commandeered local farm vehicles for ambulance purposes (Haller 2011). The task of removing the wounded from the field had been entrusted to drummer boys and musicians in the time-honoured way using stretchers and litters. Mules with baskets, called 'cacolets', strapped on to each side were also used to evacuate the wounded on stretchers. Later, a local railway was employed to remove their wounded for further care. By comparison, the French brought Larrey's system with them to the Crimea, and their ambulance service was more effective. In the American Civil War, in 1861, the armies on both sides were no better equipped than the British had been in 1853 and struggled throughout its duration to provide an adequate ambulance service for all their wounded (Bell 2009, pp. 30–42).

Sick and Injured in the Streets

In 1240, the wool porters of Florence inaugurated what eventually became the Company of the Brothers of Mercy to provide ambulance services for the city. It still exists today. They removed fever patients to a charity hospital or dead persons to a chapel on stretchers borne shoulder-high by volunteers dressed in long robes, their faces covered by hooded masks (Bell 2009, pp. 5–10). There is no record of other ambulance enterprises in the cities of Europe in the next almost 500 years. At the beginning of the eighteenth century, in Leipzig and Edinburgh, some hospitals offered porterage of the sick and injured in sedan chairs. In 1777, the Middlesex Hospital Board in London provided a horse-drawn type of wheeled sedan chair to uplift injured patients and in Manchester in 1796, the Manchester Board of Health provided a sedan chair (with a washable removable lining) to uplift fever patients to their new quarantine hospital (Bell 2009, p.15). The Chelmsford Board of Health in Essex ordered a modified cart to convey patients to hospital during the cholera outbreak of 1852. Some health boards hired wagons to take patients home (Hart 1978). It is possible that in different cities in the UK, there were second-hand cabs provided by a hospital to transport patients, but their existence is not recorded.

In 1866, Edward Barry Dalton, a former civil war army surgeon, was appointed superintendent for the Metropolitan Sanitary District in New York City and sur-rounding counties (Bell 2009, pp. 54–66). Shortly after his appointment, a cholera outbreak occurred, and in response Dalton devised a system whereby all suspected cholera cases were notified to the police who organised an immediate visit by sani-tation inspectors to confirm the diagnosis using the telegraph. They then instructed the police to summon a disinfection team in a wagon which transported the patient to a hospital which was expecting the patient. The four elements of the Dalton system were: police as first-line agents, a supporting infirmary, medical wagons on standby and dispatch of information by telegraph. The individual parts of Dalton's system would change with time, but his four principles established from this epi-sode would become the basis of modern ambulance provision. In 1869, a modern ambulance service was started by Bellevue Hospital in New York. The police were the first responders who telegraphed details about injured or ill patients who had been taken to their precinct station, and the hospital then sent an ambulance with an attendant to transport the patient to be admitted (www.emsmuseum.org 2008).

In 1862, an appeal for the provision of ambulances to bring the sick and injured to hospital was recorded in the *British Medical Journal* suggesting that hospitals should provide them (Dr Bristowe 1862, p. 389). It was largely ignored, and later in the century, ambulance development was sporadic and reactive, and in some places, there were good services but not in all. Most emergency cases requiring sur-gery were due to accidents, and these were transported in cabs, carts and stretcher arrangements. Rough handling exacerbated many injuries. A leading article from the *British Medical Journal* of 1860 tells of the famous surgeon Percival Pott, who had sustained a broken leg by falling out of his carriage. Lying on the ground, he fought off well-intentioned helpers with his stick. He refused to be moved until a door could be provided to carry him home for treatment. The case of a Mr Robert-son, a building worker, who had fallen off a scaffold fracturing his femur, is also described. He was taken in a cab to a doctor's house and from thence to hospital. On admission, he was undressed, and it was discovered that the fracture was or had be-come compound, possibly due to the unsuitable mode of carriage to hospital. It was felt that more careful handling might have avoided amputation with all its dangers (*British Medical Journal* 1860).

British society in the mid-nineteenth century was concerned about infectious illnesses and provided fever hospitals in an attempt to prevent further spread within the community. The serious problem arose of how a person suffering from a fever might be safely conveyed to hospital without infecting others en route. There be-ing no ambulances, the cab was the only transport choice for infected people who could afford it, but other options were two-wheeled handcarts, horse-drawn carts or wagons. Concerns arose that healthy members of the public could become infected in cabs which had been occupied by fever patients (*Association Medical Journal* 1856). An Act of Parliament passed in 1866 required cabbies to disinfect cabs which had carried infected persons, but this was practically unenforceable, and, in any case, there was no agreed method of disinfection specified by the act (*British Medical Journal* 1869). A penalty of a fine of £5.00 could be imposed upon any person who knowingly used a cab whilst suffering from an infectious disease (*British Medical Journal* 1866). The last cholera epidemic in London was in 1866, but, in Paris in 1882, when they suffered a cholera epidemic, its five ambulances proved inadequate, and the number was increased to 40 (*The Lancet* 1884). The Sanitary Act of 1866 placed responsibilities upon the vestries of the metropolitan districts of London to provide smallpox and fever ambulances. The process began in 1868, and by 1881, the Metropolitan Asylums Board that administered the poor-law facilities in London were providing dedicated ambulances to transport patients with infectious diseases. This body was later to organise a significant part of metropolitan London's ambulance service until 1930. Parish authorities had ambulances and disinfection procedures before 1881, but the Asylums Board's arrangements were centralised and better organised (*British Medical Journal* 1881).

In the streets, accidents were common, and it fell largely to the police authorities to organise the transfer of victims to hospitals either in a cab for those who could afford it or on two-wheeled barrows called litters. There were many different designs of these available, but Dr John Furley, one of the founders of the St John Ambulance Association, designed a modified ambulance litter which was adopted by many police forces throughout the land. Its design won a prize at the Brussels International Exhibition in 1877 (Fletcher 1979). The St John's Ambulance Association, inaugurated in 1877, initiated the first-aid training nationwide. Coalmines, iron works and railways in the northeast of England enthusiastically established workplace first-aid centres. The term, 'First Aid', was invented by the Association, and its handbook sold 28,000 copies in its first 3 years. The work of the St John's Ambulance Association became international, and by 1881, its sponsored courses were being taught all over the world, from Russia to New Zealand (Haller 1990). In 1882, in Scotland, the St Andrews Ambulance Association was formed with the same ideals. Members of the police joined first-aid classes to improve their skills in the handling of injured people.

The St John's Ambulance Brigade was established in 1887 to provide first-aid services by trained volunteers at large public gatherings. In 1888, Queen Victoria awarded it its first Royal Charter in recognition of services rendered during her golden jubilee celebrations. Outside London, the St John Ambulance Brigade invented other forms of patient transport. In Leicester, in 1892, its cycling division designed a stretcher fixed between two bicycles. In Birmingham, in 1895, a quadricycle ambulance using a stretcher between two tandems was developed, and in 1906, an unusual bicycle capable of being converted into a hand litter was introduced for country policemen (Batten 1996, p. 7). The St John's Ambulance Brigade was the first organisation in the world to organise a simulated accident exercise when it organised a 'disaster' scenario at Kings Cross station in 1899 (Fletcher 1979).

In 1882, Benjamin Howard, a contemporary of Edward Dalton, wrote in *The Lancet* proposing an ambulance service for London's metropolitan area. He was English but had emigrated to the USA, where he trained to be a doctor. His article included plans for a network of ambulances linked by telephone from police stations to hospitals similar to that existing in New York, and he and others arranged a conference for London hospital authorities to be presided over by the Duke of Cambridge (Mapother 1870, p. 78). Howard criticised the London police's wheeled litters, but perhaps this is not surprising since he was proposing a horse-drawn ambulance of his own design (Howard 1882). Howard's plans met with limited responses, and people continued to be transported to hospital as before until around 1890 when the Metropolitan Asylums Board ambulances began to transport injured people from the London streets to the nearest hospital. The last horse-drawn ambulance to be employed by them was in September 1912.

The problem for ambulance provision in the UK was funding. Parliament took the view that if local ambulances were required, then their cost was the responsibility of the local authorities. Nothing more was achieved in the nineteenth century in terms of establishing an ambulance service for London, but other cities such as Liverpool and Manchester did copy the New York example, and pressure grew on Parliament to do something about ambulance provision for the London metropolitan area. This was at a time when the small local authority area of the City of London had an efficient modern service in place, run by the police and paid for out of their police fund budget (Pollock 2013). Accidents were becoming a major problem everywhere in London with many people being killed and injured in street accidents (Hardy 1910). It took two Acts of Parliament, in 1906 and in 1914, to establish a London Ambulance Service which was a working reality by the end of the First World War.

Twentieth-Century Ambulance Services: Military and Civilian

Wars act as drivers for accelerated change in technological advancements, and the Great War brought into action modern means of dealing with the wounded. A total of 120 days after the outbreak of war, the military medical provisions for the front-line troops were debated in Parliament (Consolidated Fund Bill 1914). This Hansard report gives an excellent picture of the British army's casualty evacuation chain from the front to the hospital. A casualty was taken from the field, by stretcher or on foot, to a regimental aid post at the front, staffed by a battalion medical officer, orderlies and stretcher bearers. If necessary, he was taken from thence to an advanced dressing station approximately 400 yards behind the lines and transferred to hospital if his condition required it. Survivors were either repatriated for convalescence or returned to active service. Ambulance trains took the most seriously wounded to ports where they travelled in ambulance ships to England and thence by train to hospitals near their home towns. At the start of hostilities, there were three horse ambulances for every seven motorised ambulance, but within a year, horses had been replaced by motors.

During World War I, the British army was assisted by civilian volunteers organised by the Red Cross/St John's Ambulance collaboration as individual ambulance corps. Included among them was the First Aid Nursing Yeomanry (FANY), formed in 1907 as a female volunteer first-aid link to bring the wounded from the front line to field hospitals. Women also operated as ambulance drivers on the home front, and in 1915, they created and operated an ambulance unit in London, the Women's Reserve Ambulance (Scharff 1999, p. 91). It first saw action after a Zeppelin attack in September of that year, and in 1916, the first female-only ambulance convoy served in the British army in France. Another such civilian corps, the Munro Ambulance Corps, established in 1914 by Dr Hector Munro, included women members working as drivers on the Belgian front, several of whom were decorated for bravery. Civilian ambulance corps transported the injured from the advance dressing stations to hospitals out of the battle zone. Other volunteer ambulance corps operated under the American Red Cross, the Norton–Harjes Ambulance Corps and the American Field Service before and after the USA became involved in the war (McCallum 2008, pp. 12–14). Among the many volunteer drivers were the writers Ernest Hemmingway and Somerset Maugham and the film-makers Walt Disney and Jean Cocteau, as well as others who later achieved national and international fame in other walks of life.

After the war ended, over 300 surplus military ambulances were distributed throughout the country on a county basis and the Home Ambulance Service came into being, controlled by a central co-ordinating committee from the British Red Cross Society and the St John Ambulance Brigade in London. It was organised at county level and run by voluntary committees. Patients with the means paid for the service. For the first time, rural areas were served by an ambulance service which transported all ill and injured patients. Children and pensioners also benefitted from a patient transport service taking them to and from hospital. In 1920, they reported their first year's activities (*British Medical Journal* 1920a, b, p. 866). Major Paget, a veteran of the First World War, was its principal advisor (*British Medical Journal* 1924). By 1925, there were 375 ambulance stations in England and Wales, and the *British Medical Journal* gives the account of possibly the first major incident dealt with in the UK by a rural ambulance service. A charabanc carrying 25 people crashed in the Yorkshire Dales killing 7 people and injuring 16 others. A party of first aiders were driven in the Skipton Hospital ambulance 15 miles to Dibbles Bridge to provide services to the injured and dying on site and made four journeys to transport the victims back to Skipton (*British Medical Journal* 1925a).

After 1925, it began to be required that ambulance drivers and attendants be trained in first aid under medical supervision (*British Medical Journal* 1925b). The Home Ambulance Service later became the basis of today's service, but it should be remembered that there were also services provided by local authorities, the police, fire brigade and other voluntary organisations. Most ambulances were crewed by unpaid volunteers. Birmingham had four providers of ambulance services, the police still being responsible for transporting accident victims until 1948 (Batten 1996). In 1930, the ambulance service for London was unified under the control of the London County Council and the Metropolitan Asylum Board abolished. As a civil defence measure before the war, an auxiliary ambulance service for London was inaugurated and both services worked valiantly in the face of the blitz. After 1948, responsibilities for provision of ambulance services were apportioned to county councils as part of the National Health Act, copying the London County Council pattern.

The State of Ambulances in the UK National Health Service

Under the new National Health Service (NHS), in England and Wales, there were 146 separate ambulance services run by local authorities, one in Scotland and four in Northern Ireland (Caple 2004, pp. 18–36). There was no formal organisational structure initially, but later control was organised by either a medical officer working in a local authority health department or alternatively the local chief fire officer. Volunteer ambulance drivers continued to be used for the first 26 years of the NHS, but towards the end of this period, they had virtually all been replaced by paid employees. Their ambulances provided the most basic of facilities for patients, essentially being a 'scoop and run' service in a vehicle which was a converted van and driven by a man with only a first-aid certificate and a clean driving licence until 1968 (Caple 2004, p. 10). Gradually, ambulance drivers underwent training, and by the mid-1960s, this became a requirement for employment. The Millar Report of 1966 made extensive suggestions about training and equipment which took several years to implement. Vehicle design continuously improved and radio communications were introduced in the 1950s, beginning with amplitude modulation (AM) frequencies. These began to be replaced after 1972 by frequency modulation (FM) frequencies, and in 1974, the emergency reserve channel was introduced which allowed radio communication virtually everywhere in the UK and is still used.

In 1974, the NHS underwent a massive reorganisation with ambulance service providers being reduced from 145 to 51 for the UK. Until this time, ambulance services had been isolated and localised with no status other than as transport services for patients. The reorganisation gave an opportunity for recognition and representation of ambulance services at a national level, and regional ambulance officers, for the first time, had a say in the development of standards and increasing the professionalism of the service. Senior ambulance officers now represented the service in the Department of Health's policy and medical divisions and could influence decisions which affected the NHS at the executive level. As a consequence of the changes which followed upon the 1974 reorganisation of the NHS, ambulance workers were eventually recognised as healthcare professionals in their own right. The policy of high-quality training led to uniformity of standards for all ambulance personnel appropriate to their roles. In 1986, a nationally agreed programme of training for paramedics was inaugurated, based upon advanced training schemes which had been piloted in Wessex, Brighton, Bournemouth and Bristol. These schemes had been heavily influenced by paramedic training schemes in the USA. By 1993, ambulance technicians and paramedics, both male and female, were deployed in every front-line ambulance. The NHS underwent two more reorganisations in the twentieth century, in 1982 and in 1991, with further reduction in management bodies to 40 which by 1995 had become NHS Trusts in their own right with full independence and responsibility for their own planning and budgeting. By this time, those tasked with operational responsibilities were called metropolitan and area chief ambulance officers (Caple 2001).

The Role of Air Ambulances

The first reported air ambulance evacuation was on 16 November 1915 when a French pilot, Captain Dangelzer, flew a wounded Serbian officer out of the battle zone and later he and five other pilots evacuated 11 other casualties (Sheehy 1995). After World War I, military air transportation of battle casualties became relatively common (*The Lancet* 1933). In 1928, Australia's Flying Doctor Service began to fly doctors to ill or injured patients in Queensland and later airlifted those whose condition required it. The first use of air ambulances in the UK was in 1933 when a fisherman with peritonitis was flown from Islay in the Western Isles to Glasgow for surgical treatment (Hutchison 2009). Ever since, Scotland's Air Ambulance Service has been evacuating sick and injured patients using aircraft of different kinds from her remote communities to centrally located hospitals.

The first use of a helicopter to evacuate a wounded serviceman was in 1945 when a wounded American pilot was extracted by helicopter from the Burmese jungle (Bell 2009, p. 166). In the Korean War, helicopter evacuation became common because combat circumstances made their use obligatory, and the wounded were transferred to well-equipped modern field hospitals called mobile army surgical hospital (MASH) units where they had the benefit of the best trauma surgery available. These units have been instrumental in advancing trauma techniques which now benefit all wounded and injured people (King 2005). The American army has employed MASH units in every overseas war in which it has been involved since and has continuously improved the ambulance concept first proposed by Larrey, treating men where they lay, expeditiously removing them from harm and dealing with life-threatening injuries at a nearby substantial mobile facility before evacuating them to fixed hospitals. Variations on the MASH pattern are used by all regular armies today.

The first civilian helicopter ambulance was stationed in Santa Monica Hospital in September 1954, and helicopter ambulances were soon established in the USA. In the UK, military ambulances were available in London for emergencies in the 1970s, being replaced in 1989 by civilian helicopters. In 1987, a civilian helicopter ambulance was provided in Cornwall followed by one in Dundee 2 years later. Their success has led to the provision of helicopter air ambulances throughout the UK. They are now commonplace in most of the developed world as a means of patient transport, but there have been deaths in air crashes (*Hospital Aviation* 1989, p. 22).

Conclusion

The history of the development of ambulance services is one of continuous change with interchange of ideas benefitting successive generations. An example is seen in the pioneering work of Dr James Francis Pantridge who inaugurated the Belfast Coronary Care Scheme on 1 January 1966 using an ambulance equipped with coronary care equipment, including a defibrillator, and staffed by a doctor and coronary-care nurse (Pantridge and Wilson 1996). Research had shown that most patients died within the first hour of a heart attack and if they were to be saved, then early diagnosis and treatment, including possible use of a defibrillator, was indicated (Pantridge 1974). Pantridge's model produced such good results that it has been copied throughout the world.

The repertoire of paramedic skills continued to grow as more were trained to deal with many emergencies giving necessary resuscitation and stabilising and monitoring their patients' en route to hospital. In 1991, the London Ambulance Service provided fully equipped motorcycles for paramedics to use at times of severe traffic congestion to stabilise patients until a conventional ambulance could arrive on site. Emergency control vehicles were provided for major incidents as were emergency-equipped vehicles. There was an ongoing programme of improvement and investment to bring ambulance services to the sick and injured, and in 2001, at the initiative of one paramedic, in London, bicycling paramedics were introduced for suitable cases where heavy traffic caused access problems, and these have proved very successful and are environmentally friendly. Continuing innovation has brought 'volunteer community responders' carrying cardiac resuscitation equipment in most towns and villages in the UK, attending patients with chest pain before an ambulance can reach them. Computer-aided dispatch systems, satellite tracking and predictive analysis are new tools which have been introduced to reduce ambulance response times. Patient transport services (PTS) continue to be a feature of modern ambulance provision as are volunteer car drivers who assist in hospital outpatient transport.

The NHS has provided the testing ground for the development of an ambulance service which has been capable of responding to the needs of the sick and injured in the UK for more than 60 years, proving it to be a greatly appreciated, resilient and innovative service, responsive to changing needs. There seems to be no limit to technological innovation in health care or in electronic communication devices which can be selectively utilised for the benefit of the sick and injured who require urgent hospitalisation. Few would have foreseen trained lay volunteers using defibrillators on their neighbours to save their lives or electrocardiographic traces being sent by mobile phone by an ambulance paramedic for cardiac diagnosis in a receiving hospital. Larrey and Dalton's foundations begun 200 years ago will continue to be built upon as ambulance services strive to improve standards.

Bibliography

Anon. (1856). 'The week'. *Association Medical Journal, 4*, 275.
Anon. (1858). Leading article, 'The week'. *British Medical Journal, 1*, 74.
Anon. (1860). Leading article, 'The hygiene of surgical patients'. *British Medical Journal, 1*, 980–981.
Anon. (1866). Leading article, 'The new act on public health'. *British Medical Journal, 2*, 264–265.
Anon. (1869). 'Propagation of diseases by public vehicles'. *British Medical Journal, 1*, 103–104.
Anon. (1881). Leading article, 'The new ambulance station of the Asylums Board'. *British Medical Journal, 2*, 567.
Anon. (1884). Annotations. The ambulance service in Paris. *The Lancet, 2*, 1060.
Anon. (1900). Military Medicine in 1800. *British Medical Journal, 2*, 1870.
Anon. (1920a). The home ambulance service. *British Medical Journal, 1*, 716.
Anon. (1920b). The home ambulance service. *British Medical Journal, 2*, 866.
Anon. (1924). Home ambulance service. *British Medical Journal, 1*, 1104–1105.
Anon. (1925a). The home ambulance service. *British Medical Journal, 2*, 390.
Anon. (1925b). Development of the home ambulance service. *British Medical Journal, 2*, 1136–1137.
Anon. (1933). Air ambulances. *The Lancet, 2*, 1381.
Anon. (1989). Industry news. *Hospital Aviation, 8*(9), 22.
Batten, C. (1996). *Ambulances.* Princes Risborough: Shire Publications.
Bell, R. C. (2009). *The ambulance: A history.* Jefferson: McFarland & Company Ltd.
Bristowe, Dr J. S. (1862). Introductory lectures. *British Medical Journal, 2*, 389.
Caple, L. (2001). A concise history of ambulance services in Great Britain. *Ambulance UK, 16*, 295–297.
Caple, L. (2004). *From ambulances to almonds.* Victoria: Trafford.
Consolidated Fund (no.1) Bill. (1914). *HC Deb, 68*, cc1361–cc1457.
Fletcher, I. (1979). Aid, first and foremost: A brief outline history of the St John Ambulance Association and Brigade. *Injury, 11*(2), 104–109.
Haller, J. S. (1990). The beginnings of urban ambulance service in the United States and England. *The Journal of Emergency Medicine, 8*, 743–755.
Haller, J. S. (2011). *Battlefield medicine: A history of the military ambulance from the Napoleonic Wars through World War I.* Carbondale: Southern Illinois University Press.
Hardy, H. N. (1910). An ambulance service for London. *The Lancet, 2*, 195–197.
Hart, H. W. (1978). The conveyance of patients to and from hospital, 1720–1850. *Medical History, 22*, 397–407.
Howard, B. (1882). A hospital and accident ambulance service for London. *The Lancet, 1*, 172–176.
Howard, M. (2008). *Wellington's Doctors: The British Army medical services in the Napoleonic wars.* Stroud: The Historical Press.
Hutchison, I. (2009). The Scottish air ambulance service, 1928–48. *The Journal of Transport History, 30*(1), 58–77.
King, B. M. (2005). The Mobile Army Surgical Hospital (MASH), a military and surgical legacy. *Journal of the National Medical Association, 97*(5), 648–656.
Mapother, E. (1870). An address on American medicine delivered at St Vincent's Hospital. Dublin'. *British Medical Journal, 2*, 78.

McCallum, J. E. (2008). *Military medicine: From ancient times to the 21st century*. Santa Barbara: ABC-Clio.

Pantridge, J. F. (1974). Pre-hospital coronary care. *British Heart Journal, 36*, 233–237.

Pantridge, J. F., & Wilson, C. (1996). A history of pre-hospital coronary care. *The Ulster Medical Journal, 65*(1), 68–73.

Pollock, A. C. (2013). Ambulance services in London and Great Britain from 1860 until today: A glimpse of history gleaned mainly from the pages of contemporary journals. *Emergency Medical Journal, 30*(3), 218–222

Scharff V. (1999). *Taking the wheel: Women and the coming of the motor age*. New York: Free press.

Sheehy, S. B. (1995). The evolution of air medical transport. *Journal of Emergency Nursing, 21*(2), 146–147

Stevenson, A., & Waite, M. (2011). *Concise Oxford English Dictionary* (12th ed.). Oxford: Oxford University Press.

Williams, R. (1843). Life and works of Baron Larrey. *The Lancet, 2*, 225.

(2008). www.emsmuseum.org/virtual-museum/history/articles/398205-1869-Bellevue-Hospital-NYC.

Dr Alexander Pollock MB ChB, MPhil, MD, MRCGP, spent most of his working life beginning in 1976 in a two doctor GP practice providing 24/7 cover for his practice area spread over 64 square miles in the Scottish Borders. As such he had to deal with serious emergencies of every kind as a first responder with little or no professional support. In 2002, he took a sabbatical year off to study in the Centre for the Study of the History of Medicine at the University of Glasgow and obtained the degree of MPhil (distinction). In 2007, he retired and returned to study for the degree of Doctor of Medicine in the same department, graduating in June 2014. During the course of his research, he discovered that there was remarkably little written about the history of the development of ambulance services in the academic literature resulting into a published paper on the subject in the *Emergency Medical Journal*. Dr Pollock now works part-time as an affiliate, researching topics in the history of medicine at the University of Glasgow.

Part II
Providing Emergency Care

Chapter 3
A Strategy for Managing Quality in Ambulance Services

Mary Peters, Steve Barnard, Michael Dorrian and Kevin Mackway-Jones

Introduction and Background

While the practice of risk management and corporate governance relates to all aspects of an organisation's business and activities, the current focus within the English health service is primarily around improving quality by putting the patient first, providing an acceptable level of care, protecting patients from harm and developing a culture of transparency and openness (DH 2013a). The classification and management of risk is often considered under the headings of operational, financial and quality, and, while the management of operational and financial risks, within health-care provider organisations, are generally well established (although not always well managed), the identification, quantification and management of quality risks can be far more challenging and are of central concern to the government and public (DH 2013b).

Quality management in the context of patient care is certainly not new to the health service. Quality and, more specifically, patient safety began to emerge as a central concern from the mid-to the late 1990s, with the publication of *To Err is Human: Building a Safer Health System* (Kohn et al. 2000) in the USA. *An Organisation with a Memory* (DH 2000) was subsequently published in the UK. This resulted

K. Mackway-Jones (✉) · M. Peters · S. Barnard · M. Dorrian
North West Ambulance Service NHS Trust, Ladybridge Hall, Chorley New Road, Heaton,
BL1 5DD Bolton, UK
e-mail: kevin.Mackway-Jones@nwas.nhs.uk

M. Peters
e-mail: mary.peters@nwas.nhs.uk

S. Barnard
e-mail: steve.barnard@nwas.nhs.uk

M. Dorrian
e-mail: Michael.dorrian@nwas.nhs.uk

© Springer International Publishing Switzerland 2015
P. Wankhade, K. Mackway-Jones (eds.), *Ambulance Services,*
DOI 10.1007/978-3-319-18642-9_3

in clinical governance being developed as a framework to help drive improvements in the quality of care provided using the broad terms: efficiency, effectiveness, patient experience and clinical risk management.

Over the years, there have been many attempts to define quality in health. In 2008, Lord Darzi, as part of his review of the National Health Service (NHS) in England, created an enduring and widely accepted definition of high-quality care (DH 2008). This definition had three aspects—all of which had to be achieved:

- Care that is *clinically effective*—not just in the eyes of clinicians but in the eyes of patients themselves
- Care that is *safe*
- Care that provides as positive an *experience* for patients as possible (DH 2008)

While quality and patient safety have featured heavily in policy over subsequent years, the publication of the report into the Mid Staffordshire Trust (HMSO 2013) highlighted significant failures in quality issues and indicated that not only was there too great a tolerance of risk to patients but also that information about services was too biased towards reporting positive performance. The Berwick Report (DH 2013a) examined what changes were required within the NHS to improve patient safety, identifying that incorrect organisational priorities, systems, environmental factors and culture were contributory factors in failing to learn and in failing to protect patients from harm.

The complexity of healthcare provision and associated processes, as a risk factor, is also well documented (National Patient Safety Agency 2011). Furthermore, the uncontrolled and unpredictable environment, lack of supervision, limited information and extreme uncertainty are often suggested as factors contributing to increased patient safety risks within the pre-hospital setting (Price et al. 2013; Shaban et al. 2004; Brice et al. 2012). Stress is also considered to be a contributory factor in adverse incidents (National Patient Safety Agency 2011), with ambulance staff subjected to stressors including high workloads, shift patterns, time pressures and emotional responses to traumatic or serious incidents (Hegg-Deloye et al. 2014). Despite this, published literature on quality and patient safety within the pre-hospital setting remains limited (Price et al. 2013); with a tendency to focus more on the physical ambulance environment and the effectiveness of clinical decision making for non-conveyance decisions.

Management of Quality and Risk in Ambulance Services

The management of quality risks within ambulance services presents significant challenges due to the unique environment they operate within (Brice et al. 2012). Ambulance clinicians are often required to provide care for a diverse population in terms of demographics, levels of deprivation, medical problems and social problems. Emergency care has also been recognised as facing higher levels of risk than other areas of medicine, which is attributed to the "notion of risk and uncertainty" (Shaban et al. 2004).

The measurement of quality within ambulance services has also been traditionally limited to operational activities. In June 2011, the National Audit Office report *Transforming NHS ambulance services* stated:

Traditionally, the ambulance service has been seen primarily as a call-handling and transportation service, encompassing some aspects of patient care. (National Audit Office 2011)

The report acknowledged that ambulance services were historically more operationally focussed with the management of response times being the priority. However, the report suggested that the development of national clinical quality indicators would help shift the balance to managing the quality of patient care.

This was quickly followed by publication of "Taking Healthcare to the Patient 2: A review of 6 years' progress" (Association of Ambulance Chief Executives 2011). The report described the progress made by ambulance services since publication of *Taking Healthcare to the Patient* (Department of Health 2005) which described how ambulance services would modernise and transform to support a wider role within the health system, with care being provided closer to home. It highlighted improved response times, advances in clinical education, improved survival rates and improved patient and staff experience. The recommendations within the report included the development of high-quality clinical leadership to support the expanding clinical practice and replacement of one of the operational targets (category B calls) with a series of 11 ambulance clinical quality indicators (some of which measured clinical outcomes). The future of targets in ambulance services was to: "focus on improving patient outcomes, and balance measures of timeliness of care with measures that reflect whether the best possible clinical care has been delivered".

How Is Clinical Quality Measured and Monitored?

Clinical Audit is the mechanism through which clinical quality is measured and monitored. It has been defined by the National Institute of Healthcare and Clinical Excellence (NICE) as "a quality improvement process that seeks to improve patient care and outcomes through systematic review of care against explicit criteria and the implementation of change. Aspects of the structure, processes and outcomes of care are selected and systematically evaluated against explicit criteria. Where indicated, changes are implemented at an individual, team, or service level and further monitoring is used to confirm improvement in healthcare delivery". Some of the recent initiatives are discussed in the next section.

National Ambulance Service Audit Programmes

In April 2011, the Department of Health introduced a new series of ambulance quality indicators (AQIs) to help achieve a more balanced approach to measuring the quality of care provided. A total of 37 indicators were developed, consisting of 19 system indicators and 18 clinical indicators.

The AQIs are a specific set of indicators, audited on a whole patient cohort every month. These indicators are:

- Outcome from cardiac arrest—return of spontaneous circulation and survival to discharge
- Outcome from sinus tachycardia (ST) elevation myocardial infarction
- Outcome from stroke and *all* follow the principles of clinical performance indicator (CPI) care bundle performance measurement

Clinical Performance Indicator Care Bundles

In 2008, the National Ambulance Service Clinical Quality Group (NASCQG) developed a series of indicators on behalf of the English ambulance services. The performance information generated as a result of these audits is used by the Care Quality Commission as part of the ambulance trust Quality Risk Profile. CPI care bundle packages have been developed to cover a spectrum of pre-hospital care, such as management of asthma, hypoglycaemia, ST elevation myocardial infarction, febrile convulsions and stroke (Siriwardena et al. 2010).

Ambulance services across England use CPI care bundles to measure and monitor the quality of care given to patients. A CPI is designed to measure the elements of care that a patient may be expected to receive in the treatment of a specific clinical condition. The individual elements of a CPI may be grouped together as a "care bundle". A bundle is a structured way of improving the processes of care and patient outcomes: a small, straightforward set of evidence-based practices — generally three to five — that, when performed collectively and reliably, have been proven to improve patient outcomes (Resar R et al 2005). Specifically, CPI bundle performance can be defined as measuring the number of patients who received all the metrics/elements as defined within each of the CPIs.

As a subset of clinical audit, CPIs measure small numbers frequently to provide an indication of performance at a set point in time. Ideally, CPIs are audited at local level by clinicians with feedback given without delay to celebrate good practice and support learning needs. CPI care bundle development process has several stages. One of the most challenging aspects (after determining what clinical condition is going to be audited) is to identify those cases. This poses a particular complication for ambulance services since emergency triage tools rely on the information given remotely by the caller, which can be different from the reality. Therefore, the ideal system of case identification is by the clinicians during face-to-face contact. Once the clinical condition of interest and a method of case identification have been agreed, the next step is to decide the aspects of care that are of interest. These are the metrics that combine to make up a CPI. Metrics should be evidence based and specific to the patient cohort condition. Evidence to support interventions may come from a number of sources. The condition-specific, evidence-based elements are grouped together to form a bundle. Each metric must be delivered in order for the patient to have received the full care bundle. Occasionally, it may not be able to deliver the full bundle, for example, a patient may refuse an intervention. In these cases, provided the refusal is documented, an exception is generated which is still counted towards the patient receiving a full package of care as demonstrated in the next example (Table 3.1).

Table 3.1 Example. Asthma management: National CPI 2014/15 criteria

Short description	Percentage of asthma patients with acute or severe asthma who receive high-flow oxygen and nebulised β2 agonist bronchodilators
Evidence base	JRCALC 2013 British Guideline on the Management of Asthma 2013 Updated (Nice/Sign)
Full indicator description	100 % of patients presenting with a pre-hospital clinical exacerbation of asthma should receive high-flow oxygen therapy (C) and nebulised β2 agonist bronchodilator (A) within 5 min of assessment
Inclusion criteria	Patients with a pre-hospital clinical impression of exacerbation of asthma
Measurement method and source	Patient presenting with a pre-hospital clinical impression of exacerbation of asthma by Paramedic Emergency Service operational staff as documented on PRF
Sample	First 300 cases presenting or all if fewer
Frequency	Aligned to national CPI reporting timeline

A: directly based on category I evidence (systematic review of randomised controlled trials or at least one randomised controlled trial)

C: directly based on category III evidence (nonexperimental descriptive studies or extrapolated recommendations from category I or II evidence)

Metric		*Rationale*	*Exception*	*Data source*
A1	Respiratory rate assessed	Respiratory rates vary considerably depending on general health and activity levels. In order to establish the severity of an acute episode of asthma, it is good practice to undertake an assessment of respiratory rate	No exceptions	PRF
A2	PEFR recorded before treatment?	Using PERF assessments, attending clinicians can determine the severity of the asthma episode. PEFR can also be used as a benchmark to demonstrate patient improvement or deterioration	Patient refusal Patient unable Patient unconscious Patient does not understand Patient 5 years old	PRF

Table 3.1 (continued)

A3	SpO2 measured?	Oxygen satura-tion level assess-ments can be used by clinicians to determine the severity of the asthma episode	Patient refusal	PRF
A4	Nebulised β2 agonist administered?	The most com-monly used treat-ment for patients with asthma is Salbutamol. Salbutamol is a β2 agonist which is administered nebulised with oxygen and has a relaxant effect in the medium and smaller airway which are in spasm in acute asthma attacks	Patient refusal Contraindicated	PRF
A5	Oxygen administered?	Administration of supplemen-tal oxygen can relieve hypox-emia in moder-ate or severe exacerbations of asthma	Patient refusal SpO2 94–98% and β2 agonist contra-indicated	PRF

Care bundle for asthma (A1 + A2 + A3 + A4)

PRF patient report form, *CPI* clinical performance indicator, *PERF* peak expiratory flow rate

Quality Improvement in the Pre-hospital Arena

A peripatetic responsive service that delivers pre-hospital emergency clinical care is a challenging context in which to deliver quality improvement. Teasdale (2008) states that "Improvement is desired by everyone but delivering this however is hindered by lack of clear, widely embraced perceptions of what is encompassed within quality and how improvement can be brought about"; which describes concisely the issues faced in the ambulance arena. As described earlier, we can now measure quality through bundle reporting. This can be done on an organisation-wide basis—but this is not meaningful for the individual clinician. If a clinician can see clinical performance at an ambulance station, team or individual level, then "what needs to be done to improve" becomes more obvious as the short case suggests.

Case Study: Varying performance

The high-level CPI report shows that in the management of a specific condition, an ambulance service delivers a full package of care (the care bundle) 93.7% of the time. A breakdown report is able to describe that for the same condition over the same time period, the care bundle performance for a small area of the ambulance service is 88.7%. An individual breakdown report for two clinicians (A and B) working in that area of the service may for the same condition and time period deliver care bundle performance of 95.5% for A and 64.9% for B, respectively.

Blueprint to Quality Improvement

So what does this mean? It means that the need for improvement can be broken down to individual level. But how is that individual informed of their performance or lessons to be learned? A blueprint to quality improvement in the ambulance service is described below. This is broken down into clinical leadership education accountability and responsibility (CLEAR) and is further explained in some detail as follows:

Clinical: Leadership at Local Level

Key to the success of improving quality of care in an ambulance service is strong clinical leadership. Ideally, the clinical leaders are responsible for a team of clinicians in terms of clinical support and guidance. If mechanisms are set up to allow peer auditing by clinical leaders, the subliminal message that this is important is sent to staff. Clinicians actively performing the audit are tied in to the results and importantly the quality improvement process. It becomes meaningful to the individuals something that they are part of rather than receiving passively the results of an audit performed on them.

Leadership: There Is Never Enough Feedback

Communication through feedback is the most essential tool in a quality improvement process. If you do not tell people what they are doing well, or what could be done differently, nothing changes. Personalised feedback which celebrates success and identifies learning points is effective in consolidating improved practice. Feedback can be given by colleagues, but it is useful if it is given by a team or clinical leader as this sets the context from a general discussion to that of a learning opportunity. Similarly, feedback of success has more resonance from a clinical leader than a colleague or non-clinician as the next case will highlight.

Case Study: Trauma Care Single Limb Fracture—Main Reason for Failing a Care Bundle—Distal Pulse

The results of the CPI audit identified that there was a trust-wide issue with performing a pulse check distal to the injury site. In one sector of the Trust, the approach to remedy the situation was through several devices.

1. During one-to-one feedback sessions, senior paramedics were repeatedly told by clinicians that the intervention was performed but not written down. There was no specific space of the patient report form (PRF) to document this intervention.

2. Senior paramedics consulted with colleagues throughout the Trust, and they gained support for the recommendation that the PRF be amended to include a space for distal pulse documentation. The PRF was updated accordingly.

3. At the local level, senior paramedics continued to remind clinicians to document the intervention, and, when the new PRF became available, actively advertised that the PRF now has a specific place in which to record a distal pulse.

Output: Through one-to-one feedback, the clinician in the front line was able to receive and give feedback which changed the Trust PRF. As a result, the recording of the distal pulse has improved.

It is important that the feedback is tailored to the audience—a clinician needs individualised feedback. A senior manager will need a more strategic view. The impact of interventions in the form of annotated charts showing the outcome of changes implemented over time is a persuasive tool as is the use of statistical process control funnel plots.

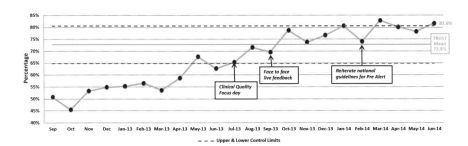

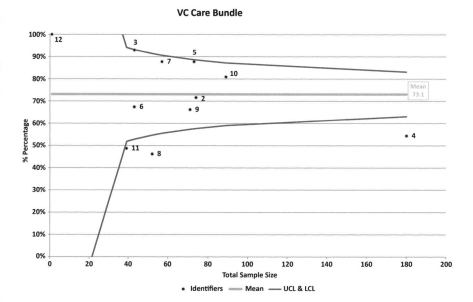

The funnel Chart as seen in the example above can be used to benchmark how ambulance services perform in comparison to each other.

Education: Plan to Improve

The clinical leader should be able to use a number of quality improvement methods to support and identify the issues causing the barrier to improving care. Through the use of collaborative quality improvement discussions, focus groups and process mapping, a series of interventions may be agreed. This may include short education packages or references to articles which are pertinent to the points of concern; all of which should be captured in a plan.

Accountability and Responsibility: At Individual Level

A quality improvement action plan serves several purposes. It provides a clear record of what the clinical teams will do to change practice, while providing a record of evidence for managers, commissioners and other stakeholders, so they know what is being done in response to the audit results. The action plan is necessary so that the implementation of actions can be monitored, and there are clear lines of accountability. Moreover, the individual has been part of the decision-making process and is responsible for ensuring that they keep to the actions they have agreed to.

Accountability and responsibility occur at service level too. The ambulance service senior leaders must show a commitment for quality improvement, and furthermore hold the responsibility for improvement. Through the receipt of regular clinical performance information, ambulance services are able to demonstrate their commitment to improving the quality of care received by patients.

Conclusion: Quality Improvement—The Next Phase

The lessons learned in developing quality improvement mechanisms across the English ambulance services are best described from the results of the Health Foundation-funded project that was run through NASCQG in 2010 (Siriwardena et al. 2014). The Ambulance Services Cardiovascular Quality Improvement Initiative (ASCQI) had two aims. The first was to improve the quality of care through the use of CPI measurement on patients with cardiovascular disease. The second was to introduce and embed the use of quality improvement techniques in the participating ambulance services. ASCQI was successful. A number of trusts showed significant improvement in the care delivered to patients; importantly, ambulance services learned and retained the quality improvement techniques which have been reinvested in other areas of work.

The introduction of CPIs across all English ambulance trusts has been successful as demonstrated through the national CPI programme. New and more sophisticated CPIs are being developed by NASCQG to supplement the current programme.

References

Association of Ambulance Chief Ambulance Officers. (2011). *Taking healthcare to the patient 2: A review of 6 years progress and recommendations for the future*. London: AACE.

Brice, J. H., Studnek, J. R., Bigham, B. L., et al. (2012). EMS provider and patient safety during response and transport: Proceedings of an ambulance safety conference. *Prehospital Emergency Care, 16,* 3–19.

Department of Health (DH) (2000). *An organisation with a Memory*. London: The Stationery Office.

Department of Health (DH). (2005). *Taking healthcare to the patient. Transforming NHS Ambulance Services*. London: The Stationery Office.

Department of Health (DH) (2008). *High quality care for all*. London: The Stationery Office.

Department of Health (DH) (2013a). *A promise to learn—a commitment to act: Improving the safety of patients in England*. London: Department of Health.

Department of Health (DH) (2013b). *Review into the quality of care and treatment provided by 14 hospital trusts in England: Overview report*. Leeds: NHS England.

HMSO (2013). *Report of the Mid Staffordshire NHS Foundation Trust Public Inquiry*. London: The Stationery Office.

Hegg-Deloye, S., Brassard, P., Jauvin, N., Prairie, J., Larouche, D., Poirier, P., Tremblay, A., & Philippe, C. (2014). Current state of knowledge of post-traumatic stress, sleeping problems, obesity and cardiovascular disease in paramedics. *Emergency Medicine Journal, 31,* 242–247.

Kohn, L. T., Corrigan, J. M., & Donaldson, M. S. (2000). *To err is human: Building a safer health system*. Washington, DC: National Academy Press.
National Audit Office. (2011). *Transforming NHS Ambulance Services*. London: The Stationery Office.
National Patient Safety Agency. (2011). *Patient Safety First: 2008 to 2010, the campaign review*. London: National Patient Safety Agency.
Price, R., Bendall, J. C., Patterson, J. A., & Middleton, P. M. (2013). What causes adverse events in prehospital care? A human-factors approach. *Emergency Medicine Journal, 30*, 583–588.
Resar, R., Pronovost, P., Haraden, C., Simmonds, T., et al. (2005). Using a bundle approach to improve ventilator care processes and reduce ventilator-associated pneumonia. Joint Commission Journal on Quality and Patient Safety, *31*(5):243–248.
Shaban, R., Wyatt-Smith, C. M., & Cumming, J. J. (2004). Uncertainty, error and risk in human clinical judgment: Introductory theoretical frameworks in paramedic practice. *Journal of Emergency Primary Health Care, 2*, 1–11.
Siriwardena, A. N., Shaw, D., Donohoe, R., Black, S., & Stephenson, J. (2010). Development and pilot of clinical performance indicators for English ambulance services. *Emergency Medicine Journal, 27*, 327–331.
Siriwardena, A. N., Shaw, D., Essam, N., Togher, F. J., Davy, Z., Spaight, A., & Dewey, M. (2014). The effect of a national quality improvement collaborative on prehospital care for acute myocardial infarction and stroke in England. *Implementation Science, 9*, 17.
Teasdale, G. M. (2008). Quality in healthcare and the quest for improvement. *Scottish Medicine Journal, 53*, 3–6.

Mary Peters is the senior clinical quality manager for the North West Ambulance Service NHS Trust. A paramedic with 20 years of experience in the NHS; Mary holds an MSc in leadership in Health and Social Care. Her specialist areas of interest include continuous quality improvement, change management and clinical leadership in health and social care. Mary is a key member of the NWAS team who received the "Closing the Gap: Ambulance Service Cardiovascular Quality Initiative" award from the Health Foundation.

Steve Barnard has worked as the head of clinical quality for the North West Ambulance Service NHS Trust since its inception in 2006. Steve was instrumental in developing ambulance clinical quality reporting and improvement systems that delivered substantive improvements in care and informed the development of national ambulance quality measures. He also leads on an annual, national ambulance audit that examines recontact rates for patients who were not transported following a 999 call. Steve also leads on End of Life Care for the ambulance sector in England and has coauthored a number of publications relating to this. Working in the NHS for 23 years, Steve is a paramedic and holds an MBA in managing in Health and Social Care.

Michael Dorrian is the risk manager for North West Ambulance Service NHS Trust. He is a member of the Institute of Risk Management and a chartered member of the Institute of Occupational Safety and Health. His previous roles include health and safety officer in a top tier COMAH site and health and safety manager for a large charity based in the North West. His specialist areas of interest include implementation of risk management frameworks and the installation risk management information systems.

Prof. Kevin Mackway-Jones was appointed as a consultant at the Manchester Royal Infirmary in 1993 and became a professor in the year 2001. He has published widely on the practice and theory of Emergency Medicine, both books (*Advanced Paediatric Life Support, Major Incident Medical Management and Support, Emergency Triage* amongst others) and academic papers. His main research interests are diagnostic strategies, psychosocial care and major incident management. Apart from consulting at the Manchester Royal Infirmary and the Royal Manchester Children's Hospital, he is also an executive medical director at the North West Ambulance Service, civilian consultant advisor to the British Army and head of the North Western School of Emergency Medicine. He is the webmaster for www.bestbets.org and the St Emlyn's Virtual Hospital through which he runs an MSc in Emergency Medicine. He was an editor in chief of the Emergency Medicine Journal from 2005–2013.

Chapter 4
Management of Emergency Demand

Bob Williams

Introduction

There is very limited academic work to explain why emergency ambulance demand continues to rise despite the changes to process, access and the public education campaigns designed to reduce it. In 2005, a bold strategic change for the ambulance service in England was outlined in the Department of Health *Taking Healthcare to the Patient* (Department of Health (DH) 2005). This proposed a raft of measures including changing the start point at which response times were calculated, reducing the number of services from over 30 to 12 and significantly up-skilling the service providers to provide a greater range of 'hear-and-treat' and 'see-and-treat' options in conjunction with significant change across the health sector.

All of this served to make the reduced number of much larger ambulance services far more efficient and effective in undertaking their core role, as illustrated in the follow-up paper *Taking Healthcare to the Patient 2* by the Association of Ambulance Service Chief Executives (2011). However, it has not slowed the rate of increase in demand for services in the emergency and urgent care setting at all. In fact, the evidence of activity levels over the past 8 years is that demand is consistently rising at an average of over 6.3 % per annum nationally demonstrated in the annual national statistics return for ambulance services (Health & Social Care Information Centre (HSCIC) 2013; Fig. 4.1).

B. Williams (✉)
North West Ambulance Service NHS Trust, Ladybridge Hall, Chorley New Road, Heaton, BL1 5DD Bolton, UK
e-mail: bob.williams@nwas.nhs.uk

© Springer International Publishing Switzerland 2015
P. Wankhade, K. Mackway-Jones (eds.), *Ambulance Services,*
DOI 10.1007/978-3-319-18642-9_4

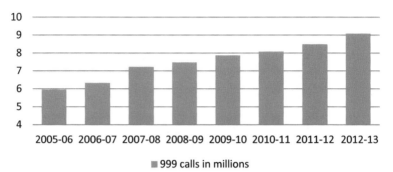

Fig. 4.1 Showing annual increase in 999 ambulance emergency calls in England. (Source: Department of Health (DH) 2012)

Evidence

So the obvious questions are why and what can be done about it? A literature review of potential contributors to rising demand for 999 ambulance services was undertaken for the National Director of Operations Group of the UK ambulance services in late 2013, a plethora of issues emerged. Table 4.1 below identifies the various factors that have been seen to be involved in the rise of service demand across the UK over the past 5 years.

This leads on to a different but challenging question—which demand are we talking about? Intellectually and strategically, we are talking about the long-term underpinning factors that affect overall demand rises for ambulance services. There are clearly many and have a number of interrelated aspects of management that can be applied (but only in cooperation with the rest of the health system and society in general). There is also the immediate tactical response to the daily demand which fluctuates hour by hour and in a longer seasonal cycle. This depends on a host of additional circumstances such as weather, hospital factors (bed availability, emergency department demand, internal processes) and primary care practices (surge created by general practitioner referrals for ambulance transport to hospital attendance).

Each of these subjects could be debated and discussed separately and there is a huge amount of anecdote and variation of opinion. However, in reality, the management of daily emergency demand is much more than an operational process matching resource to demand that is particular to the demographics, geography and funding available at local level. There are large number of documents available both in the UK (Hughes 2010; Pre-Hospital Emergency Care Council 2010) and internationally (Mcleod et al. 2010; Zuidhof 2010) that set out some general guiding principles as to how to improve the planning and management at this level.

Table 4.1 Factors impacting rise in demand of ambulance calls. (Source: National Ambulance Director of Operations Group 2013)

Population characteristics	
Age/ageing population	Disproportionate use of ambulance service by older adults (increased chronic conditions, comorbidity, polypharmacy)
	Some services report increased use by younger age groups, for example, males aged 20–29
	Falls—ageing population only accounts for small proportion of growth in demand
	Prevalence and number of long-term conditions (LTCs) increase with age
Population growth	Increased life expectancy in developed countries
	Increased birth rate and immigration in larger cities
	Growth in demand is rising faster than population growth
Population density	Demand correlated with population density
	Demand and reported inappropriate use higher in urban than rural areas
Deprivation	Demand correlated with deprivation
Car ownership	Lack of car linked to increased use of ambulance service
	Lower car ownership in urban areas and deprived areas
Migration	Lack of information/understanding of services available, lack of transport, lack of translation/interpretation
	Health risks associated with poverty and substandard housing
	Higher rates of some conditions (e.g. TB, HIV); specific health issues for refugees and asylum seekers
Homelessness	Rough sleeping and hidden homelessness increasing in England
	Greater use of ambulance service and emergency departments by homeless due to greater health needs for homeless (and also those living in substandard or overcrowded housing) and barriers in accessing primary/community care, lack of tailored services
Illness characteristics	
Triage/acuity of calls	Increasing proportion of potentially life-threatening calls
LTCs	Increasing number of people with LTC and multiple LTCs
	High comorbidity between LTC and mental health conditions
Specific conditions	Increase observed in number of calls related to breathing problems, chest pain, unconscious, traumatic falls/back injuries, psychiatric, falls (non-traumatic)
Alcohol	Alcohol-related calls account for an increasing proportion of 999 calls
Societal changes	
Changing expectations	Expectation of immediate and convenient access to assessment and treatment
	Expectation that arrival by ambulance will result in quicker treatment in the emergency department
	Changing opinions regarding what constitutes a medical emergency, and perceptions regarding what symptoms are urgent or serious
	Expectation that will receive rapid assessment and treatment from ambulance service and/or be conveyed to emergency department
Reduced social support	More people living alone and/or away from family
	More women employed, so less able to look after relatives
Technology	Increased technology and access to information—public more aware of potential symptoms
	Increased mobile phone ownership—may have lowered threshold for calling 999

The intention in this chapter is, rather, to concentrate on the strategic long-term demand for ambulance services and to promote a dialogue to share potential resolutions. So, are the UK ambulance services unique in experiencing these demand issues? Absolutely not. Not only are increases in demand being seen and discussed within the 'Anglo-American' model of ambulance services (Department of Health (DH) 2009; Queensland Ambulance Service 2007; Lowthian et al. 2011; IBISWorld 2014), this is also a point of debate in the 'Franco-German' model (Al-Shaqsi 2010) as well as further afield in Japan (Ohshige et al. 2003).

Frustratingly, two things emerge from what documentation there is. Firstly, that the underlying increase is universal with a number of similar themes emanating from socio-demographic changes of ageing and multiple illnesses combined with an urbanisation and fragmentation of communities. Secondly, that despite this being noted and documented consistently for the past 10 years across the world, there is still incredibly little clinically evidenced data for either explaining or managing the demand factors outlined above.

Analysis and Discussion

So what to do? In order to engage in a meaningful debate, some preconceived 'fixed points' and some underlying cultural absolutes will need to be set aside. Whether the ambulance service operation is based on the Anglo-American or Franco-German model, whether it is commercial or public funded, whether it operates as part of the wider emergency services system or the health system does not matter. In all cases, the demand is rising because of the factors outlined earlier in this chapter. The speed of action and combination of viable solutions may well be different depending on the system but the fundamental issues are the same. Where does the demand need to be managed? How is it managed? What are the implications?

Where does the demand need to be managed? At source would be an obvious answer. But where is that? Ideally, this is managed at the national level with a central message to the population about what the ambulance service is for and how it fits into the wider emergency services and health systems. If the messages are not clear or consistent and an expectation for inappropriate ambulance response becomes ingrained, then the first battle is lost. This certainly seems true in England at present where the underpinning principle of the National Health Services (NHS; being free at the point of entry for all) is taken as a right for everyone to call the ambulance service with the slightest ailment. This is often in addition to calling the telephone helpline service and/or calling a general practitioner.

So a question that should be asked first is what is the ambulance service for? In the Franco-German model, this is clear. The service is staffed with physicians and/or nurse clinicians and the intent is to assess, treat and discharge the majority of patients at scene. Emergency and urgent health care are treated separately with pre-established transportation regimes. In the Anglo-American model, the service is staffed with paramedics (of varying levels of education and qualification) who are responsible for initial assessment and treatment prior to referral or transportation to a hospital. The mix between emergency and urgent care is fluid. The demand on a daily basis can be managed to some extent by the enhancement of 'hear-and-treat' and 'see-and-treat' activities through increased staff education and use of triage software's, but this will not affect the underlying increases but will just change the transportation consequences.

What is clear (in the Anglo-American models of care in particular) is that demand is continuing to rise predominantly because of an increase in elderly comorbidity, increase in socio-domestic issues (alcohol and mental health driven) and increased use by the rest of the healthcare system (hospital transfers/diversions and primary care referrals). Associated with these conditions is an additional factor in England where there is significant difference in the acuity of patients between the North and South of the country due to the underlying lower health and wealth in the North (Public Health England 2011).

Which brings us back to my earlier question about what is the purpose of the ambulance service? Have we reached a point in time in the UK where a two- or three-tiered system may be required? Trauma responses are now of such small volume (in comparison to the overall activity) that they could potentially be handled by a small expansion of the hazardous area response team/urban search and rescue (HART/USAR) model that has been in place for some time with a paramedic-based skill set with dedicated trauma paramedic ambulances in order to retain competence. The significant majority of the current workload is medical, social and minor injuries and this may be best looked after by an ambulance service remodelled to mirror the principles of the Franco-German model to assess, treat and discharge at scene. This could be done by continuing to increase the education and skill sets of paramedics as well as introducing the nurse/clinician skill mix as in Europe. The third element is the 'transportation' requirements of the rest of the health system both from primary care settings and the increase in inter-hospital transfers resulting from reconfigurations of pathways of care and reductions in capacity which could be done by a separate cohort of resources, potentially as a step-up/step-down model for the other tiers.

Whatever the model is, there is a need for a national understanding with consistent messaging about what the ambulance service is for and how it fits in to the overall emergency and healthcare systems. This needs to emanate from the central government. Too much conjecture and uncertainty about the future format and function of the ambulance service that arises because of conflicting messages (around potential mergers with fire and police services and the integral role within the emergency and urgent healthcare system outlined in the Keogh report, NHS England 2013) is creating confusion. This lack of clarity is currently resulting in the ten English ambulance services determining their own visions and starting to go down very different avenues for future models of delivery. Whilst this may be entirely appropriate in terms of the local demographics, geography and health system infrastructure, it could have consequences for national cohesion in terms of education syllabus, transferability of staff and the resilience of national ambulance service infrastructure.

How can the demand be managed? Two recent papers in the UK (Strategic Health Authorities 2009; Imison and Gregory 2010) have both established the same requirement for effective management—that it can only be done in coordinated collaboration with the rest of the system the ambulance service operates within. There are two principle reasons for this. Firstly, that the paramedic skill set of the Anglo-American model is based on onward referral for the most part—thus there need to be services available for referral to. Secondly, because a significant proportion of the ambulance demand is driven by the failure of healthcare system itself (through a perceived lack of access to primary and alternative care by the public) and transport requests within the healthcare community, these must be addressed.

One simple, but potentially controversial, factor is the current use of the 999 system by the public. The intention was for 999 to be used for emergencies only. But just like the ambulance service, the term emergency has drifted far from its origins and has now become a catch-all for people who do not know how to or cannot be bothered to sort their own care issues out. So how can emergency demand be managed when an emergency is in the eye of the caller not the service provider? With the implementation of the NHS 111 number for all urgent care requirements, there is the potential to re-educate the public about the use of 999. So all health-related issues could be fielded through the 111 system (as the police are doing with 101) and only potential tri-service emergencies, such as road traffic collisions or house fires, fielded through 999. Would that delay a response to a cardiac arrest? Potentially no! When 999 is dialled, the first answer is from the telephone service operator who asks what number is being used for the call and which service is required before connecting to the ambulance service that then goes through its protocol for location, number etc. When 111 is dialled, the call is connected immediately to the health system and if cardiac arrest is identified, the local ambulance service gets the incident directly to its dispatch station with the location verified. A logical model for the ambulance service would be to manage the 111 system as the single gateway for immediate health concerns and utilise the full potential of 'hear-and-treat' as originally envisaged within *Taking Healthcare to the Patient* (Department of Health (DH) 2005). This would potentially reduce the number of immediate ambulance responses significantly.

The second element to managing the demand is what happens when the ambulance service do attend a patient. Again, the same principles of 'see-and-treat' should be explored to the full. The question for the future is can this be done with an extended paramedic knowledge base if enough alternative referral pathways are available or does it require an adjustment to incorporate the Franco-German modelling with nurse and/or clinician skill sets to treat and discharge?

What are the implications? Whatever is done to manage the demand as ambulance services see it, there will be a consequential divergence from current public expectation. This will have to be handled within the context of the overall changes to the healthcare system in England but absolutely needs a national education programme to support it.

For the past 10 years, the ambulance services in England have been developing their staff and their process to follow the principles of *Taking Healthcare to the*

Patient. This has led to something of a divergence between the established existing workforces, who are in-house 'trained' within a command and control culture, and the emerging workforce, which is Higher Education Institute (HEI) educated and asked to take individual accountability for decisions taken within the scope of their practice. A significant part of the demand management opportunity rests entirely within the ambulance service itself or more precisely with the decision-making capacity, capability and confidence of its predominant paramedic workforce. It is also a logical consequence that if the function of the ambulance service is to change, then the likelihood is that form change will follow to ensure the service is efficient and effective.

Conclusion

In England, there has been a continual rising demand for ambulance services created by a combination of elderly comorbidity, socio-domestic issues and use by the rest of the healthcare system. This, combined with a current lack of clarity from the national departments about the future role and format of the ambulance service, has resulted in a lack of public awareness and is resulting in divergence of service provision at regional level. The current operational model, skill mix and resource funding within the English ambulance service is incompatible with the public expectation and long-term activity modelling.

With the most significant change to the NHS healthcare system in a generation currently taking place, there is the opportunity for the ambulance service to play a central, constructive role in helping the transition succeed. To do that, there needs to be central recognition that the ambulance service is a fundamental part of the NHS dealing with the medical and social demand as its core business now, as it is in Scotland. The ambulance service still needs to retain a core ability to respond to trauma and major incidents coordinating and cooperating with the other blue light services, but separate from them. There needs to be open debate and honest discussion about the emergency demand requirements being made on the ambulance service so that the correct education, skill sets, operational models and functionality can be identified for the next 10 years.

References

Al-Shaqsi, S. (2010). Models of International Emergency Medical Service (EMS) systems. *Oman Medical Journal, 25*(4), 320–323.
Association of Ambulance Chief Executives. (2011). *Taking Healthcare to the patient 2: A review of 6 years' progress and recommendations for the future.* London: AACE.
Department of Health (DH). (2005). *Taking healthcare to the patients: Transforming NHS Ambulance Services.* London: Department of Health.

50 B. Williams

Department of Health (DH). (2009). *Tackling demand together: A toolkit for improving urgent and emergency care pathways by understanding increases in 999 demand*. London: Department of Health.

DH (2012). http://www.england.nhs.uk/statistics/statistical-work-areas/ambulance-quality-indicators/ambqi-2012-13/

Health & Social Care Information Centre. (2013). *Ambulance Services, England 2012–2013. National Statistics KA34 report*. London: HSCIC.

Hughes, G. (2010). The strategic health authorities' emergency services review. *Emergency Medicine Journal, 27*, 2.

IBISWorld. (2014). *Ambulance services in the US: Market research report*. NAICS 62191.

Imison, C., & Gregory, S. (2010). *Approaches to demand management: Commissioning in a cold climate*. London: The Kings Fund.

Lowthian, J. A., Jolley, D. J., Curtis, A. J., Currell, A., Cameron, P. A., Stoelwinder, J. U., & McNeil, J. J. (2011). The challenges of population ageing: accelerating demand for emergency ambulance services by older patients, 1995–2015. *The Medical Journal of Australia, 194*(11), 574–578.

McLeod, B., Zaver, F., Avery, C., Martin, D. P., Wang, D., Jessen, K., & Lang, E. S. (2010). Matching capacity to demand: A regional dashboard for Canadian ambulance services paper. *Society for Academic Emergency Medicine, 17*(12), 1383–1389.

Ohshige, K., Masako, I., Kazumitsu, N., Shunsaku, M., & Tochikubo, O. (2003). Quantitative analysis of the demand for emergency medicine in Yokohoma City, Japan. *Japanese Journal of Public Health, 50*(9), 879–889.

Pre-Hospital Emergency Care Council. (2010). *Demand analysis and tactical deployment of Ambulance Services in the National Ambulance Service Southern Region (UK)*. A report for the Pre-Hospital Emergency Care Council & the National Ambulance Service.

Public Health England. (2011). *Living longer lives*. London: Public Health England.

NHS England. (2013). *Transforming urgent and emergency care in England: Urgent and emergency care review, phase 1 report*. Leeds: NHS England.

Queensland Ambulance Service. (2007). *Audit Report*-2007. https://ambulance.qld.gov.au/index.html.

Strategic Health Authorities. (2009). *Emergency services review: Good practice in delivering emergency care*. London: NHS Office of the Strategic Health Authorities.

Zuidhof, G. M. (2010). *Capacity planning of ambulance services: Statistical analysis, forecasting and staffing*. Masters Dissertation, University of Amsterdam.

Bob Williams is the Chief Executive of the North West Ambulance Service NHS Trust, UK. Bob began his ambulance career at Northamptonshire Ambulance Service in 1985, becoming one of the country's first paramedics in 1987. He subsequently moved to South Yorkshire Ambulance Services in 1990, working in a number of training and management roles. During the early 1990s, he spent 3 years in a hospital management role where he also undertook a master's degree in Business Administration. He later returned to the ambulance service in Derbyshire as a senior manager and helped to introduce AMPDS as the first live service. Following a move to West Yorkshire as a director of service delivery (integrating ambulance operations and NHS Direct services) for 3 years, he went onto private industry as a senior consultant alongside running his own personal training/sport massage business for a year. Bob returned to the ambulance service as deputy chief executive of NWAS following the formation of the Trust in August 2006, a position he held until taking up the role of acting chief executive for the Trust in November 2012. In October 2013, Bob was appointed as the Trust's chief executive.

Chapter 5
Ethical Commissioning of Emergency Ambulance Services

Mark Docherty

Introduction

Commissioning is one of those things that is now talked about a lot in health care, but believe it or not, it is a relatively new concept in the UK. In 1988, there were only 12 mentions of the word in the UK parliament, but by 2012 there were thousands of mentions of commissioning in both chambers, and indeed, in 2011 there was a whole parliamentary Health Committee meeting to specifically investigate ambulance commissioning (House of Commons 2011). So something has changed in the last 25 years to make ambulance commissioning such an interesting subject—why is this? The answer lies in how we define ambulance commissioning, because unlike the process of contracting, the process of ambulance commissioning is a cycle that begins much earlier by identifying the urgent and emergency health needs of our population or community and designing the pathways of care provided by an ambulance service that will meet the needs of those people. By specifying and procuring ambulance services within the resources available, commissioning ensures that people get good care in the context of appropriate models and frameworks, and this also needs to take account of ethical considerations.

Ambulance commissioning therefore will involve a process of priority setting, which may involve deciding how best to make future investments, or in some cases may involve deciding which services are no longer being provided.

For the ambulance service in the UK, demand has generally gone up by around 5 % a year for the last 20 years, and although some of this increase can be explained by the population demographics (e.g. an increasing elderly population), this does not explain the total increase, and some of the rise may simply be that people expect

M. Docherty (✉)
West Midlands Ambulance Service NHS Foundation Trust,
Millennium Point, Waterfront Way, Brierley Hill, DY5 1LX Dudley, West Midlands, UK
e-mail: mark@docherty.info

© Springer International Publishing Switzerland 2015
P. Wankhade, K. Mackway-Jones (eds.), *Ambulance Services,*
DOI 10.1007/978-3-319-18642-9_5

to be able to call for an ambulance whatever health need they have. Ambulance commissioners therefore have a difficult task of ensuring there is the right amount of resource to meet the population needs for this service against the wider challenges of ensuring that any spend on health care maximises the population health. This can be a hugely difficult thing to do and probably explains why commissioning gets so much attention at the highest level. Each day, there are numerous ethical dilemmas that we face, and this chapter looks at ways in which we can ensure that ambulance commissioning is set in the context of being ethical, and some of the principles and processes that move this from an impossible to a manageable process.

Ethical Ambulance Commissioning

All healthcare commissioning involves allocating resources, and this becomes particularly challenging as resources become more limited. Challenging ethical dilemmas arise when trying to prioritise which services get funded compared to others. Ambulance commissioning occurs in this complex environment of competing priorities and ethical dilemmas, so let us think what some of those situations might be:

- *Should we fund services for people who do not need them?* If we know that a large number of people use an ambulance service for health needs that are not life-threatening or for which there are other services available, should we still provide an ambulance for them? What if there is no ambulance available to attend to somebody in cardiac arrest because the ambulance is attending somebody that does not have a life-threatening or urgent health need?
- *How do we measure the impact of investment in ambulance services?* If we can understand the health outcome delivered by an emergency ambulance service, then we can compare the investment against other health interventions. For example, where a person has major trauma, we know that an emergency ambulance getting to them quickly with a skilled paramedic able to deliver life-saving interventions before rapidly transferring the patient to a major trauma centre has significant health benefits that justify investment in this type of service. On the other hand, it is likely that a young person with a cough who calls an ambulance service to take them to hospital because they have no transport is unlikely to result in a significant return on the health investment in the ambulance service, and it may be argued that this service should not be provided.
- *How do we prioritise investment in ambulance services against other investment priorities?* Even where a service is clinically effective, there are still decisions that have to be made to prioritise investment. For example, if we think that we need to invest money to improve the emergency ambulance service for people with mental health crisis, how do we make the case against the investment needed to improve care for premature babies?

The decisions and priorities that need to be made by ambulance commissioners and providers of ambulance services can be complex. In addition, we have the added political dimension of services that are in the public eye; who, for example, wants to see an elderly lady who has fallen in the street wait for an ambulance even if arguably the wait may not result in further harm to her condition. In this case, an economic evaluation would not come up with the right answer because public opinion would simply not support a slow response to such need.

Because the public highly value an emergency service and will generally want a rapid response if they need it, politicians see this as an important issue to address and apply arbitrary targets for emergency ambulances to respond to a person in need. In the National Health Service (NHS) in England, for example, there is a target for the time taken for an ambulance to arrive at a person who is deemed to have a life-threatening (red 1) or potentially life-threatening (red 2) condition; the current target states that in 75 % of these cases, an emergency ambulance should arrive at the patient within 8 min. This creates some interesting discussion, as 8 min is an arbitrary target that would be of little benefit in a situation of cardiac arrest where the patient would almost certainly have died if they waited that long; and even where a quick response is needed, why is a target set at 75 % (what about the other 25 % of patients)? The reality is that many of the people that fall into this category of urgency do not end up being this severely unwell or injured, but in England this single measure of performance has become the political target that determines whether an ambulance provider is successful or not. The fact that some of the target measures are of dubious scientific rigour creates a dilemma for ambulance commissioners who often invest large amounts of resource to hit the targets, often at the expense of other interventions. But even if these targets are not clinically necessary, the public tell us often that equally they do not like waiting a long time for an ambulance to arrive. So even if these targets are arbitrarily set and create as many dilemmas as they solve and consume huge amounts of resource without being clear on how this benefits patient outcomes, patients often just would not accept a slower response, and this creates a dilemma.

Ensuring Ethical Priority Setting and Resource Allocation

Because healthcare resources are diminishing on a relative basis in most countries in the world, this means that not everybody can have what they need and want all of the time, so we need to find ethical ways to help us decide what services get funded and which ones do not. Much of the research and the rationale for priority setting is set in the context of acute medicine where some of the measures and evidence are at a much greater state of maturity. Hospitals, for example, have been measuring patient outcomes for many years, but the application of these methods to the commissioning of an emergency ambulance service can be more complicated because the information may simply not be available.

There are two fundamental ethical principles that should be applied to the commissioning of an ambulance service in all situations (adapted from Dworkin 2002). The first is that every person's life has intrinsic value and should be considered with equal concern, where every life matters irrespective of any other factor that is present. The second is that people have responsibility for their own life, but in delivering an ambulance service, we should not be judgemental about the life choices that a person has made, and care should be delivered equally to all people. Assuming we can accept the above principles, then there are initially three things that need to be considered in an ethical sense when making decisions about the commissioning of an emergency ambulance service:

1. *Doing good (utility)*—cost-effective analysis is a way in which we identify priorities for investment, and health commissioners will often look to maximise the effect of their investment, and this is referred to as allocative efficiency (allocative efficiency is a term used to describe a system where there is an effort to maximise health-related utility per unit cost).

   Health economists would advocate a mechanism of ensuring the greatest return on investment. A quality-adjusted life year (QALY) is an example of this approach and is used by the National Institute for Health and Care Excellence (NICE) in the UK. Where QALY is used as the only mechanism of prioritising resource allocation, this can disadvantage people with a limited life expectancy, such as those who are elderly or who have a long-term condition. It is also unfair for those people who have less to gain from particular interventions, such as people with disabilities. This approach can be applied to many ambulance interventions—for example, a service that is able to effectively treat people with stroke, myocardial infarction and trauma is likely to score high on this measure. It is more difficult to apply this type of methodology to an elderly person with dementia who has fallen, for example, as the ambulance intervention on its own is unlikely to increase the person's life expectancy or quality of life.

   When considering 'doing good', it is also important to consider the wider benefits of an intervention. In the UK, for example, a review of major trauma care was undertaken, resulting in the development of improved pre-hospital care by ambulance services and the introduction of specialist major trauma centres. When evaluating the impact of the resource allocation, whilst QALYs were used, a wider impact assessment was undertaken, including the extent to which a person became independent and contributed to economic self-sufficiency. So when we assess the benefit of an ambulance service in economic terms, we need to consider the impact on patient survival and the impact on their quality of life and other benefits that patients may consider important. We also consider how an ambulance service contributes to the overall efficiency of health care; and in the UK ambulance services are increasingly the first point of contact for people who have urgent care needs, making the service a critical part of a system to ensure that people get to the right place of care and treatment in a timely manner.

2. *Being fair*—because of the inherent problems of resource allocation being based on utility (doing good) alone, in ambulance commissioning we often focus atten-

tion as much on the issue of the process of allocation being fair (referred to in the literature as 'distributive justice'). Being fair is important to people and our evidence would suggest that members of the public are satisfied that we may do less good overall, so long as we deliver in a fair way. An example of this would be the delivery of an emergency ambulance service to urban and rural areas. The speed of an ambulance response is important where a person has a life-threatening condition, but should the time that a person has to wait for a response differ in urban and rural areas? Those people that advocate a fair system of delivery might suggest that the speed of response should not be affected by the urban or rural nature of where the emergency situation is, even if providing the same speed of response requires a relatively more expensive resource allocation in the rural areas. Other people might argue that it is fair for people to wait longer in areas where population density is sparse but might argue that clinical outcomes should not be adversely affected, so this might require a different response model in order to maintain the highest level of care whilst awaiting the arrival of an emergency ambulance.

3. *Doing the right thing*—initially this might be encompassed by the principles of 'doing good' or 'being fair', but there is a slightly different perspective that ambulance services need to consider from an ethical perspective. If a service cannot be justified on the basis of 'doing good' or 'being fair', it can often be considered on the basis of 'doing the right thing'. Consider, for example, a person who is injured whilst committing a crime, but whose injury is not life-threatening. We could argue that treating them takes resource away from people who are genuinely sick, but ambulance services need to treat people in a way that is non-judgemental by 'doing the right thing'.

   There are other situations where it is clearly not cost-effective to provide a service, but some situations or services conflict the need to assess purely on the grounds of 'doing good' and 'being fair', and this is particularly the case for emergency services where there is a legitimate view that civilised societies should fund services to save lives despite the cost. This concept often causes some professionals working in pre-hospital emergency care a dilemma, as clearly in a cash limited healthcare system this creates an imbalance between 'doing good' and 'being fair'. If massive amounts of resource were allocated to services that delivered to a more than likely futile outcome then it is likely that people would question the rationale for this.

So the three factors that we have to consider when prioritising investment in our ambulance services are often creating opposing tensions and differing priorities or ethical dilemmas, but there is a fourth consideration for emergency services that I describe as 'being seen to be doing the right thing'. There are some emergency situations where you have to provide help irrespective of whether it is cost-effective, fair, or the right thing to do. For example, think of a situation where a person has been trapped in a collapsed building; ambulance services will often commit large amounts of resource to the safe recovery of a single person, and often at huge risk to the people involved in the rescue, and this continues even where the chances of a person's survival become increasingly low. Jonsen (1986) refers to this as the 'Rules of Rescue', where the public expect a significant response as there are often identifiable people in tragic circumstances.

'Being seen to be doing the right thing' doesn't always conflict with the other principles, as the cost of saving an identifiable person from death in many instances may be minimal; for example, where an ambulance service provides cardio-pulmonary resuscitation to a person in cardiac arrest, the benefit of saving a life is so great and the cost of doing so low, that the action dictated by the 'Rules of Rescue' happens also to be the most cost-effective one, but the measure is undertaken initially without immediate consideration for the cost-effectiveness. Let us then consider a different example where a person has jumped from a high building and is still alive on the road below. We know that the likelihood of survival is low, but the principle of the 'Rules of Rescue' is that despite this, we are likely to mobilise significant resource to try and help the person who is severely injured. There is therefore a human mindset that suggests that the logical and rational approach implied in the cost-effectiveness analysis is disregarded when a person's life is threatened, and in certain situations there is a duty to help a person irrespective of the cost-effectiveness ratio, or the likely chances of the person's survival.

'Being seen to be doing the right thing' provides an added dimension to the principles of ethical commissioning. Think, for example, of the resources that are put in place for severe emergencies, such as major trauma teams, and the Helicopter Emergency Medical Services (HEMS). These services are often provided at great cost, and albeit they are not always universally funded through public money, arguably have a cost that might not be supported if a pure cost-effectiveness case were to be applied. The fact that people are willing and keen to support services that are not the highest priority when assessed by a cost-effective analysis suggests that human nature must be taken into account in order for any proposals to be seen to be ethical and be acceptable to the public.

When delivering ambulance services, people can take the view that all services should be provided in all situations regardless of cost; however, in a cash-limited healthcare system, it can be difficult to reconcile this public pressure of being seen to be doing the right thing, against the reality of maximising health benefit from limited resources. Ambulance service providers and commissioners should consider this from the context of a 'prudent person' (Dworkin 2002) who would spend money on health care throughout their life, but would generally set this against other things that they value, such as education and housing. Ambulance commissioners, acting as an Agency for a 'rational person', might forego some heroic treatment of dubious value in return for more certain benefits of other ambulance interventions.

The three principles of *'doing good', 'being fair' and 'doing the right thing',* set against the context of 'being seen to be doing the right thing' highlight the challenges that commissioners have and the fact that it is unreasonable to procure an ambulance service on the basis of a single principle. For example, if resources are allocated on the basis of identified need, then other principles such as cost-effectiveness may be ignored, but if we allocate resource simply on the basis of 'doing good', then a large proportion of ambulance resource will be allocated to those incidents where we know there is a positive health benefit and would fail to consider how the allocation of this resource negatively impacts on those people with less immediate needs. 'Doing good', 'being fair' and 'doing the right thing' are often priorities that pull in opposite directions, so the challenge for ambulance services and commissioners is to ensure that there is a balance between the three and to consider other principle of 'being seen to be doing the right thing' in order to reach a decision.

Ensure Fair Decision-Making: Involving Clinicians, Patients and the Public

When we commission an ambulance service whilst recognising the need to 'be fair', it is also important 'to be seen to be fair', and whilst this may seem pedantic, the process of fair decision-making is probably as important as the principle of 'being fair' and is probably harder to achieve than might appear at first sight.

There have been many attempts in the UK and around the world to provide principles and rules to support decision-making. In the UK, for example, we have a number of strategic documents that set out the direction of travel for the delivery of an effective ambulance service, but these are often fairly abstract in nature and on their own are unlikely to result in effective action. Work undertaken around the world by Sabik and Lie (2008) suggests that strategy needs to be interpreted by expert national bodies to consider how it would be implemented in specific interventions, and in the UK we have a number of expert bodies providing the necessary expertise in translating policy, such as the Association of Air Ambulances (AAA), the Association of Ambulance Chief Executives (AACE) and the Ambulance Commissioners Network (ACN).

Even where due process is followed to reach a decision when we are commissioning emergency services, the result is often that we are faced with irreconcilable conflicts that are not easily resolved, and we need to consider how these irreconcilable decisions can be managed. Recent moves in the NHS in England have been to involve clinicians in the commissioning process for emergency ambulance services through clinical commissioning groups (CCGs). Clinicians often view conflicts in a different way to administrators as they are used to these difficult dilemmas in their everyday practice, and Heath (1999) refers to this as the 'oscillating gaze' where the seemingly impossible scenario is managed to a successful conclusion by considering all aspects of the dilemma. Experienced paramedics are often faced with logically irreconcilable conflicts in everyday practice, for example, incidents that require them to prioritise treating one patient before another, or in major disaster situations possibly not treating some patients at all. Whilst commissioning an emergency ambulance service might be slightly different in the focus (e.g. the needs of a particular patient vs. the needs of society in general), clinicians often cope well in these seemingly impossible situations where mysteriously all aspects of the dilemma are considered to ensure that where possible, a satisfactory decision or compromise is reached. Clinical commissioning is a concept that is relatively new in the UK, but having experienced clinicians involved in decision-making and priority setting is crucial to a successful outcome and recognising and nurturing people with such skills is critical to a successful outcome.

Clinicians are integral to both the formulation of commissioning policy and the implementation of it. This creates something of a double-edge sword, where on the one hand, the patient needs to be assured that the paramedic will take the best decisions on behalf of an individual patient, but on the other hand, it will need to consider scarcity in considering that decision.

Priority setting will always be liable to ethical dilemmas; so, systems need to be robust to be sure that where there is likely to be some challenge of the decision or there is no universal consensus, there are systems that legitimise the decisions or give legitimacy to the outcome. Because not all decision-making will be taking place in a perfect world, and there is a potential for decisions to be tainted by value judgements or indeed conflicts of interest, then it is important that any decisions on prioritisation or disinvestment are taken in a fair way, with 'procedural justice'; that is to say, that even if somebody does not agree with the decision that has been taken, they are able to see that it has been undertaken in a fair and just way.

Resource scarcity creates problems for emergency services, particularly in the context of reducing resource, increasing demand, and increasing expectations from service users and the public. Funding reductions for publically funded emergency services are a reality in many countries around the world during the current global recession. In previous years, informal mechanisms of priority setting were the norm and went largely unchallenged, but due to the size of the current fiscal challenge in many areas, politicians are supporting the concept of explicit priority setting (Sabik and Lie 2008).

Involving clinicians in priority setting can help align conflicting priorities, but involving the public and service users is an equally important priority for the delivery of effective ambulance services for a number of reasons:

1. It is a good thing to do—service users have a right to be consulted about their health services, and it enables them to be empowered and in control of the services they use. It is also a good way by which traditional ambulance services can be challenged to deliver more patient focused care.
2. It is socially and politically important—involvement of members of the community will help to support the proper use of ambulance services by invigorating the social and civic responsibilities of participants, and ensuring ambulance services have strong local voices back into the communities they serve.
3. It can ensure ambulance services focus on improvement of care and outcomes— service users can be used as a means to a better end and allow consideration of the patient voice in how the service is delivered.

Involving service users that are representative of all service users can be a challenging process. On average in the NHS in England, a person will have the need to phone 999 for an ambulance about once every 6 years, so many people have little experience or knowledge of the service until the point at which they need it, and at this point they may be unwell and experience the service for a relatively short time in the overall pathway of their care. Even after experiencing the service, many people may not have a particularly strong view of the service, unless it has not met their expectations, so it can be challenging to involve the public in this process; however, even where people do not have much experience as a service user, it is still important that their views on fair decision-making processes are sought.

Some ambulance services have a concern that individual stakeholders may attempt to exert undue influence, but where stakeholders form into organised groups, they can be particularly useful in ensuring that the voice of people who are traditionally marginalised have their voice heard; London Ambulance Service, for example, has a very effective Patient's Forum that work closely with the service and commissioners to ensure a strong patient and public voice.

Whether it is patient involvement in ambulance service prioritisation or wider public involvement in decision-making, it is likely that a decision will have greater legitimacy if it has the patient and public acceptance of the fairness of the decision-making process. Patient and public involvement cannot simply be a token gesture as this would create mistrust and cynicism, and the following examples need to be avoided:

1. Agenda setting—the ambulance provider or commissioner controls the terms of the debate and may also prevent some issues being discussed. For example, service users are consulted about the closure of some ambulance bases, but are not given information on all viable options, or selectively include service users' views.
2. Preference shaping—the ambulance provider or commissioner influences people's thoughts, desires and perceptions. For example, they do not seek to influence a decision to close some ambulance bases because they believe that the only valid evidence for decision-making is the official or clinical view of the ambulance service provider.
3. Decision-making the ambulance provider or commissioner informs people of a decision that has already been taken, but refers to this as consultation. For example, the ambulance provider or commissioner takes a decision to close an ambulance base and seeks simply to inform the service user.

For some services that people do not use very frequently, such as ambulance services, the public may not want to be involved in decision-making, and very often they would rather leave difficult decisions to professionals who have access to a wider range of information and are able to assimilate this more readily. For a service that is not used regularly by most people, there can be a tendency for more informed patients to come forward as user representatives, and this in itself can cause some difficulties as the regular service user becomes professionalised into the role, and this questions whether such people could be representative of the community as a whole.

Despite the challenges of involving service users and the public, it is important that there is a legitimate process through which their valuable input can be sought in a proactive and constructive way.

Conclusion

Urgent and emergency ambulance services are a critical part of the pre-hospital infrastructure and are held in high regard with service users and the public. These services are working in a challenging climate where decisions on priority setting have to be made within an ethically acceptable framework. Commissioners and ambulance service providers need to ensure that services that are in place are effective (do good) and that decisions on priority setting are fair. For ambulance services, however, there is an additional consideration of services that 'do the right thing', so service providers and commissioners need to take into account these three, often conflicting priority considerations when specifying the model of ambulance response.

Making decisions about the priorities for investment can be a difficult process, and although there are numerous scientific and rational approaches that can be used to reach a decision, the fact that ambulance services are in the public arena means that not only must the decisions be fair but also the process of decision-making needs to be transparent and accountable. For ambulance services, the principles of ethical commissioning using a scientific and rational approach will not always reach a conclusion on priority setting, and two additional factors need to be taken into account when reaching decisions.

Firstly, clinical engagement is critical. Paramedics and other clinicians are very skilled in clinical priority setting and have the ability to make decisions when there are competing clinical priorities. Involving paramedics and other clinicians in the wider health system will enable difficult priority setting decisions to be made in the context of ethical dilemmas.

Secondly, it is important to involve patients, service users, and the public to ensure that the patient voice is considered and to ensure that the decision-making process is seen to be fair, adding a greater legitimacy to any decisions that are proposed. Ensuring good levels of public and service user engagement ensures that difficult decisions made by commissioners of ambulance services have a legitimacy that justifies the reasonableness of the decision and the decision-making process.

A triangulated approach to ethical decision-making for urgent and emergency ambulance services will provide the most ethically robust process for priority setting. Using a rational and scientific approach, engaging paramedics and other clinicians, and involving service users and the public are critical to successful decision-making.

Bibliography

Dworkin, R. (2002). Sovereign virtue revisited. *Ethics, 113*(1), 106–143.
Heath, I. (1999). Uncertain clarity: Contradiction, meaning and hope. *British Journal of General Practice, 49*(445), 651–657.

House of Commons. (2011). Transforming NHS Ambulance Services. *House of Commons Committee of Public Accounts, Forty-sixth Report of Session 2010–2012.*

Jonsen, A. R. (1986). Bentham in a box: Technology assessment and health care allocation. *Law, Medicine and Health Care, 14,* 172–174.

Sabik, L. M., & Lie, R. K. (2008). Priority-setting in health care: Lessons from the experiences of eight countries. *International Journal for Equity and Health, 7*(1), 4.

Mark Docherty is the Director of Nursing, Quality and Clinical Commissioning for West Midlands Ambulance Service NHS Foundation Trust. West Midlands Ambulance Service NHS Foundation Trust serves a population of 5.36 million people covering an area of more than 5000 square miles in the heart of England, and as the region's emergency ambulance service responds to around 3000 '999' calls each day. Mark has previously been the ambulance commissioner for London Ambulance Service, and in 2013 gave evidence to the House of Commons Health Committee on urgent care that led to the Urgent and Emergency Services Second Report (2013).

Part III
Context of Emergency Care

Chapter 6
Organisational and Professional Cultures: An Ambulance Perspective

Paresh Wankhade, James Radcliffe and Geoffrey Heath

This chapter concerns the nature of culture within the emergency services and ambulance service in particular and how this impacts on the prospects for reform. It considers the different types of culture(s) with reference to organisational and professional cultures, their place within recently published policy statements on reform of the National Health Service (NHS) as a whole and the ambulance services in particular, the role of subcultures and how changing performance frameworks may help change these cultures. Notwithstanding the methodological and conceptual limitations of any such analysis, the exploration of the culture(s) in the ambulance service is an important topic for academic enquiry.

The concept of organisational culture is one that has come to the forefront of studies of organisational change in recent years with a concern that structural changes on their own are inadequate as a means for reform. As was noted by Morrill (2008, p. 16), the 'emergence of organizational culture frameworks that emphasised organizations as systems of meanings and symbols' has been an important contribution to the discipline. The development of theories and research around new institutionalism reinforced this move with ideas around the 'cultural-cognitive' nature of organisational structures (Scott 2004). These developments became an important focus of attention for the study of organisational change in the 1990s. This

P. Wankhade (✉)
Edge Hill Business School, Edge Hill University, Room B204, Ormskirk, L39 4QP, UK
e-mail: Paresh.Wankhade@edgehill.ac.uk

J. Radcliffe
Faculty of Health Sciences, Staffordshire University, Blackheath Lane, Stafford, ST18 0AD, UK
e-mail: jim.radcliffe@staffs.ac.uk

G. Heath
Keele Management School, Keele University, Keele Staffordshire ST5 5BG, UK
e-mail: g.heath@keele.ac.uk

© Springer International Publishing Switzerland 2015
P. Wankhade, K. Mackway-Jones (eds.), *Ambulance Services,*
DOI 10.1007/978-3-319-18642-9_6

was centred on an awareness of the heterogeneity of organisational cultures and the consequent concern with the role of subcultures which could subvert established ways of doing things (Scott 2004, p. 29).

But why is reform claimed to be needed? Paradoxically, while the public's attitude towards the ambulance personnel remains very positive (as life savers), evident from the high scores in various Ipsos MORI polls, the social context of ambulance service delivery is rapidly changing. The massive cuts in public spending coupled with fundamental structural changes brought about by the coalition government (Health and Social Care Act, 2012) has led to new thinking about how to deliver services by doing 'more for less'. With the government aiming for up to £20 billion of efficiency savings in the NHS by the end of 2014–2015, the National Audit Office (NAO 2011) expects the ambulance service to play a part in achieving these savings by identifying a minimum of 4% efficiency savings (around £ 75 million per year) within its budget. The abolition of the primary care trusts (PCT) and their replacements by the new clinical commissioning groups (CCGs), along with the emergence of private ambulance providers such as *Arriva,* are fundamentally changing the emergency care landscape in the UK (Halsall et al. 2013). This calls for a clearer understanding of the role and contribution of the ambulance service in the UK, in addition to identifying more efficient ways of delivering the service.

However, this interest in organisational culture is problematic as there has been a proliferation of definitions of 'culture' and how it impacts upon organisational behaviours. Browaeys and Price (2008, p. 9) note that 'one can never use the term culture without being obliged to give a range of definitions that contradict each other'. Schein (1985, p. 17) defines organisational culture as a 'pattern of shared basic assumptions that was learned by a group as it solved its problem of external adaptation and internal integration; and that has worked well enough to be considered valid, and therefore-to be taught to new members as the correct way to perceive, think, and feel in relation to those problems'.

There has also been the development of both descriptive and normative approaches to the study of organisational culture. The latter has aimed at being influential in the creation of a more efficient and effective health service. In addition, Konteh et al. (2010) have contended that there are two major approaches to the conceptualisation of organisational culture. First, culture is a 'metaphor' for an organisation, and it is something that it is. This enables an organisation to be distinguished from others in their social behaviour as a cultural construct. Second, culture as an 'attribute' which is more concerned with what an organisation has, such as technology, physical environment and products.

Most definitions do, however, recognise the socially constructed nature of a phenomenon that is expressed in terms of patterns of behaviour. Notwithstanding the disagreements over the precise definition of organisational culture, it is generally agreed that culture operates in layers. Thus, Schein's (1985) identification of a pluralistic dimension of culture operating at three distinct levels is a useful framework of analysis and is supported in the literature (Wankhade 2012; Sackman 1992). For Schein, at the first level are the 'artefacts' which are the most visible manifestations of culture, including the rewards, rituals and ceremonies, and are concerned with the observational patterns of behaviour (e.g. green uniform for ambulance crews) which might be both easy to identify and difficult to decipher. At the next level are the espoused 'beliefs and values' which may be used to justify particular behavioural patterns (e.g. speed of ambulance response). At the third level are the 'assumptions' which are the real and largely unconscious beliefs and expectations held and shared by individuals. A shared value or belief is transformed into a shared assumption (e.g. uniformed emergency service vs. emergency health service).

Role of Occupational Cultures and Organisational Behaviour

Studying and understanding organisational cultures within emergency services are becoming popular. Waddington (1999) argued that police culture has been used to explain and condemn a broad spectrum of policing practices, often being presented as single, monolithic and static. This view is contested by many researchers who point out the differences within and variety of policing subcultures (Westmarland, 2008.). There are meaningful differences between the ways in which organisations display a public image and in their day-to-day practices. In a study of police subcultures, Barton (2003, p. 357) concluded that the failure of successive attempts at police reform results from a deeply rooted occupational culture suspicious of the purpose of reform, resulting in cynicism among rank and file officers. More recently, Loftus (2010) has argued for the durable nature of the police culture and has shown how it has survived the period of transition, with officers displaying remarkable continuity with older patterns of behaviours and values. He concludes that the police culture endures because the basic pressures associated with the police role have not been removed, thus questioning the increasingly accepted view that orthodox conceptions of police culture no longer make any sense. Wankhade (2012) came to similar conclusions in his analysis of ambulance cultures.

The effectiveness of a wide variety of organisations, including health care, has been linked with the culture of the organisation (Cameron and Freeman 1991; Wilderom et al. 2000; Davies et al. 2000). There is some intuitive appeal in the proposition that organisational culture may be a relevant factor in healthcare performance. However, the possible relationship between culture and performance is not conclusively established since both 'culture' and 'performance' as variables are conceptually and practically distinct (Scott et al. 2003a, b; Wankhade and Brinkman 2014). International evidence linking culture to organisational effectiveness is rather mixed (Mannion et al. 2005; Gerowitz et al. 1996), and it is suggested that a major cultural transformation needs to be secured alongside structural and procedural change to deliver expected improvements in healthcare performance and quality (DH 2000).

While this should lead to some caution in its application, it has still been proposed that using organisational culture as a means to improve health care can bring positive results and changing organisational culture is now a familiar prescription for health sector reform in the UK (Ferlie and Shortell 2001; Scott et al. 2003a). This holds that the NHS and its constituent organisations possess a discernable culture, and the nature of such cultures has some bearing on performance and quality (Wankhade 2012; DH 2001; Mannion et al. 2005). Cultural change is thus high on the government agenda and involves all elements of cultural and organisational changes. Key aspects are said to include empowering front line staff to use their skills and knowledge to develop innovative services, with more say in how services are delivered and resources are allocated, and changing the NHS culture and structure by devolving power and decision-making to front line staff led by clinicians and local people (DH 2001, p. 2).

The final report of the Mid Staffordshire NHS Foundation Trust Public Inquiry (Francis Report 2013) into the patient deaths there emphasised the need for organisations to create and maintain the right culture to deliver high-quality care that is responsive to patients' needs and preferences. The report made 290 recommendations designed to change this culture to make sure patients come first, creating a common patient-centred culture across the NHS. The King's Fund (2013) identified two distinct messages coming out of the Francis Report:

- A transformation of systems, leadership and organisational culture is needed throughout the NHS, if the lessons of the Francis Inquiry into the shocking failings of care at Mid Staffordshire are to be learned and acted on.
- The leadership of the NHS at a national level needs to create the conditions in which high standards of care are delivered consistently, setting clear goals and standards for improving quality and patient safety, and providing the means for staff to deliver these goals within available resources.

This is particularly evident within the discourse that has emerged from organisations such as the NHS Institute for Innovation and Improvement (now contained within the NHS Improving Quality website). Their concern with organisational culture was evident in areas such as the patient experience (http://www.institute.nhs. uk/patient_experience/guide/the_importance_of_organisational_culture.html) and in the development of programmes concerned with improving quality of service delivery through programmes such as 'Organising for Quality and Value: the fundamentals of Quality Improvement' (http://www.institute.nhs.uk/quality_and_value/ organising_for_quality_and_value_/organising_for_quality_and_value_homepage. html). It was also evident in the development of the 'NHS Leadership Qualities Framework' where change was seen as a central part of the programme.

In a recent statement on the NHS website concerned with the implementation of 'High Quality for All, now and for Future Generations', Sir David Nicholson stated 'After what feels like 10 years of the NHS...obsessing about structures and systems, culture is starting to get the profile it deserves' (http://www.england.nhs. uk/2013/07/26/david-nicholson-2/). Indeed, as Konteh et al. (2010) argued in relation to the public inquiry into children's heart surgery at the Bristol Royal Infirmary, the recommendations 'highlighted a number of cultural shifts seen as necessary to transform the NHS into a high-quality, safety-focused institution, one that was sensitive and responsive to the needs of patients'. Consequently, they saw that there was an 'increasing interest' in 'managing organizational cultures as a lever for improving quality of care' (p. 111).

Professional Cultures

One of the most significant issues within the health service as a whole has been that of working within a multi-professional organisation in which there is the potential for conflict between professions of various standing and those areas of activity which have little or no recognised professional status. As Salhani and Coulter (2009, p. 1221; see also King and Ross 2003) have argued:

> All health professionals (including medicine) are relentlessly pursuing their various professional projects by seeking state sanction for consolidated and/or expanded professional boundaries and for the right to, or defence of, self-governance, particularly in reference to professional work autonomy.

For this reason, newer occupational groups, such as podiatrists and radiologists, have sought professional recognition. Within emergency services, paramedics provide the most interesting example of this move towards professional status and the consequent cultural change that this brings. Reference can be made to the well-established literature around the role of professionalisation as a process which entails the socialisation of individuals into a role and set of behaviours deemed appropriate by the professional body (Hyde 2010; Hyde et al. 2012; Hassard 1993; McCann et al. 2013; see Butcher and Stelling 1977; Hayden 1995). Even within the well-established professional groups, recent challenges have emerged which have led to questions about how to better socialise professionals into the positive roles and ethics supported by the professional body. A recent report for the Royal College of Nursing (Rejon and Watts 2013, p. 1) aimed to explore 'strategies to support positive socialisation of nurses'.

This has implications for paramedics since the ambulance service, by the nature of contact with the patients, is at the front line of the NHS, and it is incumbent upon the service to examine its own clinical and leadership practices. Blaber and Harris (2014) have recently argued for a development of the clinical leadership for the paramedics as 'sine qua non' of ambulance professionalisation. The Keogh Review on urgent and emergency care (NHS England 2013, p. 29) called for a system-wide transformation of emergency care services with carefully developed clinical standards and outcome measures.

Changing the Culture in the Ambulance Service

In recent years, there has grown a concern with the establishments of concepts such as the 'learning organisation', in which there is an emphasis on change as a constant within organisations. The culture required to cope with such an environment is open to regular training and personnel development (Garcarz 2003). This is particularly pertinent within the context of changes within the health service sector where there has been a continuing emphasis on an increased need for professional development and changing roles as identified by the Keogh Review (NHS England 2013). However, Wankhade and Brinkman (2014) argued that 'top-down' attempts to bring about cultural transformation might not necessarily find traction at the frontline on account of constant pressure of meeting performance targets against ever increasing demand of 999 calls.

The renewed calls for the professionalisation of ambulance staff have led to a debate around the requirement for changes in training and culture. First et al. (2012) contend that

> for paramedics to truly take on board professionalism in its entirety, engagement with their professional body needs to take place to better effect the self-determination of the profession and greater engagement with its future direction.

This concern is also evident internationally, where the development of paramedics as a profession is taking place as skills expand and health services demand a greater degree of care on site by emergency services. For example, O'Meara (2009, p. 2) has commented on the situation in Australia where the role of cultural change is seen as a key to this development:

> …language and symbolism are important when we refer to ourselves as paramedics and professionals rather than some of the older terms that some of us have memories of, such as drivers, bearers and officers.

In a study of the UK paramedics, Woollard (2009, p. 4) has also noted that

> teaching professionalism is about changing knowledge, skills and attitudes. Professionalism in action is also a cultural issue, consisting of collective as well as personal beliefs, attitudes and inter-professional behaviour.

Lack of clinical educational and training of the ambulance workforce is still seen as a big cultural challenge (Wankhade 2011a, b; Siriwardena et al. 2010). There is also a growing recognition that a huge amount of paramedic training is about trauma and very little of what they actually deal with when they go out on the road is about trauma (AACE 2011). There needs to be further debate about shifting the educational base from local training with a broader emphasis on diagnostic medical assessment and greater standardisation (Lovegrove and Davis 2013, p. 9).

Although progress is being made in the areas of education and training and staff appraisal, the report found that the ambulance workforce still, by and large, feels undervalued and wants more support, which is partly linked to response time targets and in particular the unintended consequences that too narrow a focus can produce, at least some of the time (Wankhade 2011b; Wankhade and Brinkman 2014).

Extending Roles and Skills of Ambulance Personnel

Consequently, it is necessary to continue to develop the skills of ambulance crews and paramedics through increasingly high-level education and training, which will enable them to engage in safe and reliable triage activity on the scene, as well as provide a wider range of treatment (Ball 2005).

This argument may be linked to the development of emergency care practitioners (ECPs), dating from 2000, which entailed a major redesign of the paramedic's role (Ball 2005). Cooper et al. (2004) established that the emerging role of the ECP, whilst somewhat unclear at that time, focused on advanced assessment and patient management skills. They explored the ways in which the role of the ECP varied from that of the ambulance paramedic. Notably, ECPs were significantly more likely to treat the patient at the scene and less likely to have the patient conveyed on to an accident and emergency (A & E) department. ECPs and stakeholders agreed that the additional training received by the ECP had improved their clinical practice.

The 'treat-and-refer' approach likewise entails staff with enhanced skills being trained to use new protocols regarding non-transportation of patients. Compared to routine practice, there were similar conveyance rates to A & E, but a longer time was spent at the scene with more in-depth assessment. Patient satisfaction ratings were similar or greater (Snooks et al. 2005). However, there were some safety concerns and issues around managing change in introducing complex clinical and service developments. Interestingly, again there were difficulties in persuading some patients that they did not need to go to A & E.

Mason et al. (2007a) report on a project to evaluate appropriateness, satisfaction and costs in respect of ECPs, compared to more traditional approaches to emergency care. They concluded that the availability of ECPs was affecting positively ways of working locally and the reconfiguration of service delivery. The use of ECPs led to reduced attendances at A & E and reduced admissions, shorter episode times and higher levels of satisfaction. Furthermore, they suggest, although cautiously, that the ECP model of service delivery may give cost savings, particularly with regard to reducing operational costs, although a significant investment in training expenditure was also required.

In reviewing patients' experiences of care provided by ECPs compared to traditional ambulance practitioners, Halter et al. (2006) found that the care provided by ECPs was considered equal or considerably better, especially with regard to 'thoroughness of assessment'. Fewer patients dealt with by ECPs were being conveyed to A & E, suggesting that utilising ECPs to explore alternative treatments improves patient satisfaction. Similarly, Mason et al. (2007b) examined the benefits of a scheme by the South Yorkshire Ambulance Service, utilising extended skills practitioners to assess and, if necessary, treat older people with minor injury or illness in the community. They concluded that the initiative provided a clinically effective alternative to standard ambulance transfer in such cases, although they had some concerns regarding the level of inter-agency cooperation required and the amount of training and operational costs.

For Gray and Walker (2008), advanced practitioners who can assess and treat at the point of access are increasingly important and can provide potentially significant cost savings to the NHS. Bevington et al. (2004) even argued that the development of new roles at Essex Ambulance Service, including ECPs, contributed to the rapid improvement in performance there from zero to two stars. Given the apparent efficacy of these approaches, a key question which then arises is: Do the organisational cultures of ambulance services support these developments?

The NAO (2011) acknowledged that research suggested advanced practitioners could achieve potential reductions in transfers of patients to A & E of 30% by treating them at the scene and that some services were, or were considering, using them in ways which make the most appropriate use of their greater skills. In most ambulance services, however, they concluded that, in practice, they

> ...have tended to use advanced practitioners alongside paramedics, without targeting them where they can have the greatest impact on conveyance rates. (NAO 2011, p. 31)

Moreover, it is claimed that

> evidence suggests that the call categorisation system currently in use in most services is not sophisticated enough to direct practitioners to the most suitable calls. (NAO 2011, p. 31)

This raises some doubt as to whether the changing role is being fully adopted and, in turn, whether it is supported by the organisational culture.

A New Beginning?

A concern with both organisational and professional culture is evident within a number of reports emerging from government and government agencies since the first national ambulance review, *Taking Healthcare to the Patient: Transforming NHS Ambulance Services* (DH 2005), which revealed an interest in the changing skill mix of emergency service personnel. The review emphasised organisational culture and the role of leadership. It noted that while ambulance services were effective at delivery of services, there had been a lack of investment in the development of staff from ambulance crews through to managers (para 3.11, p. 10). The report further noted that there was a need to develop the skills of front-line staff to deliver a more effective service:

> It is evident that investing in the clinical development of front-line ambulance staff can yield significant returns for the whole health economy in terms of increased patient satisfaction and improved health outcomes.

The ambulance review also noted that a key to the transformation of the culture of the organisation was through improvements in leadership, in line with the NHS commitment to the Leadership Qualities Framework. However, a key area for development was in line with the developing role of community paramedics and ambulance crews as a whole (Sect. 4 Vision, pp. 14–24). This would entail a change in education and training to increase their role in dealing with cases on-site and reducing the emphasis on transferring patients to a hospital or other healthcare service. Consequently, a key recommendation of the report was that 'ambulance services should provide an increasing range of other services eg: in primary care, diagnostics and in health promotion' (p. 23). This obviously represented a key challenge to the existing culture of many parts of the ambulance service.

As a result of this emphasis on the role of leadership in changing cultures, the NHS Ambulance Chief Executive Group followed up the publication of 'Taking Healthcare to the Patient' with research into how this could be effectively implemented. This resulted in 'Taking Healthcare to the Patient 2' which reviewed progress on achieving the key recommendations of the original government report (for a full discussion of results, see AACE 2011).

The NAO with its concerns for efficiency of services noted that the internal cultures of different ambulance services throughout England and Wales 'inhibited the take-up of some good practice' (NAO 2011, p. 7 para 11). In particular, they held that this had led to variations in the application of performance measurement criteria, making it difficult to compare performance around the country and thus resulting in a lack of consensus about 'what "good practice" looks like'.

A major review of the development of the role of paramedics was also conducted by the service delivery and organisation (SDO) network (NHS Confederation 2011a, b). As with the development of the Department of Health's thinking and increasingly that of ambulance services and the paramedic's professional body, this report into the work of critical care paramedics (CCPs) in South East Coast Ambulance NHS Trust (SECAmb) placed an emphasis on still further increasing the skill base and educational level of key staff (see Newton 2011 for full discussion about the role of CCPs in relation to ECPs). However, the creation of this specific group of paramedics may result in a particularly significant subculture emerging within the ambulance service at a time when a change in culture is already being consolidated during a period of significant change.

The discussion in the previous section and the underlying message of improving culture is consistent with the findings of the recent ambulance review (AACE 2011, pp. 76–77) which suggested that improving staff satisfaction remains a challenge for the ambulance service. The report highlighted the need to create organisations that look, feel, behave and deliver differently (AACE 2011, p. 77). Earlier, the Bristol inquiry reported that cultural characteristics of the NHS fostered a climate where dysfunctional behaviour and malpractices were not effectively challenged (Kennedy 2001). It also highlighted the collection of fragmented, loosely coupled, and self-contained subcultures existing at Bristol Infirmary (Weick and Sutcliffe 2003). This is also support by the Francis Inquiry Report (2013).

But the question remains what is the 'right' culture of patient care? The next issue of identifying the culture(s) within organisations and further changing it is far more complex. There is a growing academic debate (Price 2006; Heath and Radcliffe 2007, 2010) around the contention that the continuous focus on performance targets based on response times reinforces the risk averseness in the organisation.

It also goes against the widening skills agenda to which we alluded earlier in the chapter, and it is opportune to emphasise again here the potential clash of cultural values which stress speed to scene and to A&E and those which stress enhancing skills and the wider role of the paramedic. Recent evidence (Wankhade and Brinkman 2014; Wankhade 2011a; Wankhade 2011b; Radcliffe and Heath 2009; Cooke 2011) further highlights improving the culture in the ambulance service in transforming the service into a professional and clinically led organisation. However, recent changes to the performance measurement regime (Cooke 2011), at least, seem supportive of the broader role (see Heath and Wankhade 2014).

Classification of Ambulance Culture

There have been relatively few attempts to classify ambulance cultures. However, Wankhade (2012, p. 383), in an ethnographic study of an NHS ambulance trust in England, identified three distinct occupational subcultures using Schein's (1996) typology:

- The 'operator' culture represented by the frontline crews (paramedics and technicians) who respond to all emergency 999 calls
- The 'engineering' culture represented by the Emergency Medical Dispatch Centre (EMDC) staff—call takers and call dispatchers where all 999 calls are received and vehicles dispatched to the scene of an emergency
- The 'executive' culture representative of the chief executive and the senior executive team

The study reported a variety of assumptions and values were held by the different occupational cultures described above and found that that there is no 'single' ambulance culture but 'multiple' cultures in the chosen organisation. Respondents spoke as members of their occupational 'tribes', each with its own assumptions, values and beliefs which was further reinforced by their specific attitudes towards performance (Schein 1996, p. 385).

Empirical evidence on attempts to manage and change ambulance culture is only just emerging. Wankhade and Brinkman (2014) in their empirical study of a large ambulance trust in England studied the culture change process and documented several unintended consequences of the culture change process (see also Harris and Ogbonna 2002). These included:

- 'Ritualisation' of the culture change effort to an annual/periodic ritual
- 'Hijacked process' which results in the change of founding ideals of the change programme
- 'Cultural erosion' in which the espoused ideals are eroded by subsequent events
- 'Cultural reinvention' denoting espousal of attitudes and behaviours which, while appearing new, merely camouflage continued adherence to the old culture
- 'Ivory tower' cultural change reflecting cultural change plans which are either divorced from organisational reality or cannot produce meaningful implementation

- 'Inattention to symbolism' that is inherent in that organisation
- 'Behavioural compliance' with the long-term aim of changing the values, beliefs and assumptions of the employees, who go through the motions, but their basic attitudes remain unchanged

McCann et al. (2013, p. 772) make a similar argument about a lack of meaningful synthesis of senior level institutional entrepreneurship and an informal lower-level form of institutional work as contributing towards the lack of success of the ambulance professionalisation project. The authors concluded that changes suggested at the top do not necessarily have a buy-in at ground level which creates disconnect within the organisation. In the absence of a clear ownership, direction and acknowledgment of occupational identities, attempts to bring cultural change are particularly likely to lead to unintended consequences (Wankhade and Brinkman 2014). It follows that there is a case for a systematic identification and evaluation of the risks of such effects during the planning stage, as well as during and after the application of culture change initiatives (Hatch 1993). It is thus important to have meaningful results for efforts to bring about cultural change along with structural and procedural reforms, while taking into account the potentially perverse consequences of such a process along with its overall impact on the employees.

Conclusion

Despite the efforts made by ambulance trusts to culturally transform themselves into a clinically driven workforce, they may still be perceived primarily as a male-dominant 'call-handling and transportation service' (NAO 2011) dealing with life-threatening emergencies around trauma (e.g. road traffic collision), severe breathing problems and cardiac arrest (Kilner 2004; Lendrum et al. 2000; Cooper 2005). McCann et al. (2013) talk about the challenges in transforming ambulance personnel from a 'blue collar trade' into healthcare professionals.

Lack of clinical educational and training of the ambulance workforce is seen as a big cultural challenge. Vestiges of the old command and control culture, accompanied by a tendency to blame (Commission for Health Improvement, CHI 2002), hierarchical and top-down management style, and resistance to change and being risk-averse (NHS Modernisation Agency 2004) are some of the factors cited historically within the ambulance service as barriers to such a transformation (McCann et al. 2013). Woollard (2006, p. 5) in presenting details of different paramedic training initiatives around the UK highlights considerable variations in the 'length, content and academic level of the associated educational programmes'. The NAO (2011) suggests moves towards developing ECPs may be going into reverse due to retention issues. Their utilisation might be further affected by the impact of austerity measures.

Ambulance leaders (AACE 2011) continue to argue about the need to professionalise the work force by transforming the work culture. Attempts on the part of the ambulance services to fully integrate within the wider NHS have also been hindered by the confusion which still prevails within its members about the core values and mission of the service (NHS Confederation 2011a, b). Recent evidence also suggests that some of the issues concerning ambulance performance targets including unintended consequences might have their origins in the underlying cultures in the ambulance service (Radcliffe and Heath 2009; Wankhade 2011b, 2012).

McCann et al. (2013, p. 771) recently argued that the senior level professionalisation strategy has so far had limited traction due to power issues and other institutional priorities/pressures. They contend that the College of Paramedics is growing in significance, but other powerful organisations such as the Association of Ambulance Chief Executives (AACE) are centrally involved in influencing the behaviour of paramedics and imagining the future directions of travel for the paramedic profession. They conclude:

> Short-term priorities of hitting targets, winning care contracts, and 'keeping the show on the road' are far more important to NHS trusts than any aspirant long-term projects such as paramedic professionalization. Institutional work in such a setting is necessarily less about trying to change organizations and institutions, and more about maintenance. (McCann et al. 2013, p. 772)

To conclude, we agree that the complexity of culture as an amorphous concept, subject to various local contingencies, makes it difficult to reform or change. We have also reflected on the changing role and identity of ambulance personnel and the conflict between professional cultures and management objectives, including lack of organisational resources. Moreover, the contrasts between the complexity of culture and the necessarily simple nature of performance measurement have significant policy and practice implications. All these issues make this a fascinating topic to study and research.

Bibliography

Association of Ambulance Chief Executives. (2011). *Taking healthcare to the patient 2: A review of 6 years' progress and recommendations for the future, June 2011*. London: AACE.

Ball, L. (2005). Setting the scene for the paramedic in primary care: A review of the literature. *Emergency Medical Journal, 22*, 896–900.

Barton, H. (2003). Understanding occupational (sub) culture—a precursor for reform: The case of the police service in England and Wales. *International Journal of Public Sector Management, 16*(5), 346–358.

Bevington, J., Halligan, A., & Cullen, R. (2004). From zero to hero. *Health Service Journal, 114*(5916), 26–27.

Blaber, A., & Harris, H. (2014). *Clinical leadership for paramedics*. Berkshire: Open University Press.

Browaeys, M.-J., & Price, R. (2008). *Understanding cross-cultural management*. Harlow: FT/ Prentice Hall.

Butcher, R., & Stelling, J. (1977). *Becoming professional*. London: Sage.

Cameron, K., & Freeman, S. (1991). Culture, congruence, strength and type: Relationship to effectiveness. *Research in Organizational Change and Development, 5*(1), 23–58.

Cooke, M. (2011). An introduction to the new ambulance clinical quality indicators. *Ambulance Today, 8*(1), 35–39.

Cooper, S. (2005). Contemporary UK paramedical training and education. How do we train? How should we educate? *Emergency Medicine Journal, 22,* 375–379.

Cooper, S., Barrett, B., Black, S., Evans, C., Real, C., Williams, S., et al. (2004). The emerging role of the emergency care practitioner. *Emergency Medicine Journal, 21,* 614–618.

Commission for Health Improvement (CHI). (2002). What CHI has found in ambulance trusts. www.healthcarecommission.org.uk/NationalFindings/National. Accessed 25 March 2008.

Davies, H., Nutley, S., & Mannion, R. (2000). Organizational culture and health care quality. *Quality in Health Care, 9*(2), 111–119.

Department of Health (DH). (2000). *An organisation with a memory: Report of an expert group on learning from adverse events in the NHS. Chaired by the Chief Medical Officer.* London: Department of Health.

Department of Health (DH). (2001). *Reforming emergency care: First steps to a new approach.* London: Department of Health.

Department of Health (DH). (2005). *Taking healthcare to the patient: Transforming NHS ambulance services.* London: Department of Health.

Ferlie, E., & Shortell, S. (2001). Improving the quality of health care in the United Kingdom and the United States: A framework for change. *Milbank Quarterly, 79*(2), 281–316.

First, S., Tomlins, T., & Swinburn, A. (2012). From trade to profession—the professionalization of the paramedic workforce. *Journal of Paramedic Practice, 4*(7), 378–381.

Francis, R. (2013). *Mid Staffordshire NHS Foundation Trust Public Inquiry. Final report.* London: The Stationery Office.

Garcarz, W. (2003). *Make your healthcare organisation a learning organisation.* Abingdon: Radcliffe Medical Press.

Gerowitz, M. B., Lemieux-Charles, L., Heginbothan, C. & Johnson, B. (1996). Top management culture and performance in Canadian, UK and US hospitals. *Health Services Management Research, 9*(2), 69–78.

Gray, J., & Walker, A. (2008). Avoiding admissions from the ambulance service: A review of elderly patients with falls and patients with breathing difficulties seen by emergency care practitioners in South Yorkshire. *Emergency Medicine Journal, 25,* 168–171.

Halsall, J. P., Wankhade, P., & Cook, I. (2013).The big society in a time of crisis—The impact on public health. *Illness, Crisis and Loss, 21*(4), 341–353.

Halter, M., Marlow, T., Tye, C., & Ellison, G. (2006). Patients' experiences of care provided by emergency care practitioners and traditional ambulance practitioners: A survey from the London ambulance service. *Emergency Medicine Journal, 23,* 865–866.

Harris, L.C, & Ogbonna, E. (2002). The unintended consequences of culture interventions: A study of unexpected outcomes. *British Journal of Management, 13*(1), 31–49.

Hassard, J. (1993). *Sociology and organization theory: Positivism, paradigms, and postmodernity.* Cambridge: Cambridge University Press.

Hatch, M. J. (1993). The dynamics of organizational culture. *Academy of Management Review, 18*(4), 657–693.

Hayden, J. (1995). Professional socialisations and health education preparation. *Journal of Health Education, 26*(5), 271–278.

Heath, G., & Radcliffe, J. (2007). Performance measurement and the English ambulance service. *Public Money and Management, 27*(3), 223–227.

Heath, G., & Radcliffe, J. (2010). Exploring the utility of current performance measures for changing roles and practices of ambulance paramedics. *Public Money and Management, 30*(3), 151–158.

Heath, G., & Wankhade, P. (2014). A balanced judgement? Performance indicators, quality and the English ambulance service; some issues, developments and a research agenda. *The Journal of Finance and Management in Public Services, 13*(1), Early cite.

Hyde, P. (2010). Changing relationships between health service managers: Confrontation, collusion and collaboration'. In J. Braithwaite, P. Hyde, & C. Pope (Eds.), *Culture and climate in health care organizations.* Basingstoke: Palgrave MacMillan.

Hyde, P., Granter, E., Hassard, J., McCann, L., & Morris, J. (2012). Roles and behaviours of middle and junior managers: Managing new organizational forms of healthcare. NIHR Service Delivery and Organisation Programme: HMSO.

Kennedy, J. (2001). *Learning from Bristol: Public inquiry into children's heart surgery at the Bristol Royal Infirmary 1984–1995*. London: Stationery Office.

Kilner, T. (2004). Educating the ambulance technician, paramedic, and clinical supervisor: Using factor analysis to inform the curriculum. *Emergency Medicine Journal, 21,* 379–385.

King, N., & Ross, A. (2003). Professional identities and interprofessional relations: Evaluation of collaborative community schemes. *Social Work in Health Care, 38*(2), 51–72.

King's Fund. (2013). *Patient-centred leadership: Rediscovering our purpose.* London: The King's Fund.

Konteh, F. H., Russell, Mannion, & Huw T. O. Davies (2010). Understanding culture and culture management in the English NHS: A comparison of professional and patient perspectives. *Journal of Evaluation in Clinical Practice, 17,* 111–117.

Lendrum, K., Wilson, S., & Cooke, M. W. (2000). Does the training of ambulance personnel match the workload seen? *Pre-hospital Immediate Care, 4*(1), 7–10.

Loftus, B. (2010). Police occupational culture: Classic themes, altered times. *Policing and Society: An International Journal of Research and Policy, 20*(1), 1–20.

Lovegrove, M., and Davis, J. (2013). Maximising paramedics' contribution to the delivery of high quality and cost effective patient care, High Wycombe: Buckinghamshire New University.

Mannion, R., Davies, H., & Marshall, M. (2005). *Cultures for performance in health care.* Berkshire: Open University Press.

Mason, S., O'Keefe, C., Coleman, P., Edlin, R., & Nicholl, J. (2007a). Effectiveness of emergency care practitioners working within existing emergency service models of care. *Emergency Medicine Journal, 24,* 239–243.

Mason, S., Knowles, E., Colwell, B., Dixon, S., Wardrope, J., Gorringe, R., et al. (2007b). Effectiveness of paramedic practitioners in attending 999 calls from elderly people in the community: Cluster randomized control trial. *BMJ, 335,* 919.

McCann, J., Granter, E., Hyde, P., & Hassard, J. (2013). Still blue-collar after all these Years? An ethnography of the professionalization of emergency ambulance work. *Journal of Management Studies, 50*(5), 750–776.

Morrill, C. (2008). Culture and organization theory. *Annals of the American Academy of Political and Social Science, 619,* 15–40.

National Audit Office (NAO). (2010). *Major trauma care in England. HC 213, Session 2009–2010.* London: The Stationery Office.

National Audit Office (NAO). (2011). *Transforming NHS ambulance services.* London: The Stationery Office.

Newton, A. (2011). Specialist practice for paramedics bright future? *Journal of Paramedic Practice, 3*(2), 58–61.

NHS Confederation. (2011a). *Critical care paramedics: Delivering enhanced pre-hospital trauma and resuscitation care: A cost-effective approach.* London: NHS Confederation.

NHS Confederation. (2011b). *An involving service: Ambulance responses in urban and rural areas.* London: NHS Confederation.

NHS Modernisation Agency. (2004). *Driving change: Good practice guidelines for PCTs on commissioning arrangements for emergency ambulance services & non-emergency patient services.* London: NHS Modernisation Agency.

NHS England. (2013). *Transforming urgent and emergency care in England: Urgent and emergency care review. Phase 1 Report.* Leeds: NHS England.

O'Meara, P. (2009). Paramedics marching toward professionalism. *Journal of Emergency Primary Health Care, 7*(1), 1–3.

Price, L. (2006). Treating the clock and not the patient: Ambulance response times and risk'. *Quality and Safety in Health Care, 15,* 27–30.

Radcliffe, J., & Heath, G. (2009). Ambulance calls and cancellations: Policy and implementation issues. *International Journal of Public Sector Management, 22*(5), 410–422.

Rejon, J. C., & Watts, C. (2013) *Supporting professional nurse socialisation: Findings from evidence reviews*. London: Royal College of Nursing.

Sackman, S. A. (1992). Culture and subculture: An analysis of organisational knowledge. *Administrative Science Quarterly, 37*(1), 140–161.

Salhani, D., & Coulter, I. (2009). The politics of interprofessional working and the struggle for professional autonomy. *Nursing, Social Sciences and Medicine, 68*(7), 1221–1228.

Schein, E. H. (1985). *Organisational culture and leadership*. San Francisco: Josse-Bass.

Schein, E. H. (1996). Three cultures of management: The key to organizational learning. *Sloan Management Review, 38*(1), 9–20.

Scott, W. R. (2004). Institutional theory: Contributing to a theoretical research program. In K. G. Smith & M. A. Hitt (Eds.), *Great minds in management: The process of theory development*. Oxford: Oxford University Press.

Scott, J., Mannion, R., Davies, H. T. O., & Marshall, M. (2003a). Implementing culture change in health care: Theory and practice. *International Journal for Quality in Health Care, 15*(2), 111–118.

Scott, J., Mannion, R., Davies, H. T. O., & Marshall, M. (2003b). Does organisational culture influence health care performance? *Journal of Health Service Research Policy, 8*(2), 105–117.

Siriwardena, A. N., Donohoe, R., & Stephenson, J. (2010). Supporting research and development in ambulance services: Research for better health care in prehospital settings. *Emergency Medicine Journal, 27*(4), 324–326.

Snooks, H., Kearsley, N., Dale, J., Halter, M., Redhead, J., & Foster, J. (2005). Gaps between policy, protocols and practice: A qualitative study of the views and practice of emergency ambulance staff concerning the care of patients with non-urgent needs. *Quality and Safety in Health Care, 14*, 251–257.

Snooks, H., Evans, A., Wells, B., Peconi, J., Thomas, M., Woollard, M., et al. (2009). What are the highest priorities for research in emergency prehospital care? *Emergency Medicine Journal, 26*(2), 549–550.

Waddington, P. A. J. (1999). Police (canteen) sub-culture: An appreciation. *British Journal of Criminology, 39*(2), 287–309.

Wankhade, P. (2011a). Emergency services in austerity: Challenges, opportunities and future perspectives for the ambulance service in the UK. *Ambulance Today, 8*(5), 13–15.

Wankhade, P. (2011b). Performance measurement and the UK emergency ambulance service: Unintended consequences of the ambulance response time targets. *International Journal of Public Sector Management, 24*(5), 384–402.

Wankhade, P. (2012). Different cultures of management and their relationships with organizational performance: Evidence from the UK ambulance service. *Public Money and Management, 32*(5), 381–388.

Wankhade, P., & Brinkman, J. (2014). The negative consequences of culture change management: Evidence from a UK NHS ambulance service. *International Journal of Public Sector Management, 27*(1), 2–25.

Weick, K. E., & Sutcliffe, K. M. (2003). Hospitals as cultures of entrapment: A re-analysis of the Bristol Royal Infirmary. *California Management Review, 45*(2), 73–84.

Wilderom, C., Glunk, U., & Maslowski, R. (2000). Organizational culture as a predictor or organizational performance. In N. M. Ashkanasy, C. P. M. Wilderom, & M. F. Peterson (Eds.), *Handbook of organizational culture and climate*. Thousand Oaks: Sage.

Westmarland, L. (2008). Police cultures. In T. Newburn (Ed.), *Handbook of Policing* (pp. 253–280). Cullompton: Willan.

Woollard, M. (2006). The role of the paramedic practitioner in the UK. *Australian Journal of Paramedicine, 4*(1), Article 11.

Woollard, M. (2009). Professionalism in UK paramedic practice. *Australian Journal of Paramedicine, 7*(4), Article 9.

Prof. Paresh Wankhade is a Professor of Leadership and Management at the Edge Hill University Business School. He has done his PhD in Ambulance Performance & Culture Change Management from the University of Liverpool, UK. He is the founder editor of the *International Journal of Emergency Services* (an Emerald group Publication) and is recognised as an expert in the field of emergency management. He has chaired special tracks on leadership and management of emergency services at major international conferences including the annual European Academy of Management (EURAM) Conference, British Academy of Management Conference and Public Administration Committee (PAC) Conference. His research and publications focus on analyses of strategic leadership, organisational culture, organisational change and interoperability within the emergency services. His publications have contributed to inform debates around interoperability of public services and challenges faced by individual organisations. His latest book on *Social Capital, Sociability and Community Development* explores these issues including the state of the pre-hospital care in eight selected case study countries (UK, USA, China, India, Bangladesh, Japan, Netherlands and South Africa) around the world.

Dr. James Radcliffe is a fellow of Staffordshire University based in the Faculty of Health Sciences. He was trained as a political scientist and lectured primarily on Health and Public Policy. His publications cover a wide range of topics in particular (1991) *The Reorganisation of British Central Government* and (2000) *Green Politics: Dictatorship or Democracy?* Since 2006 he has published a number of articles on the UK ambulance service and the role of performance indicators with Geoffrey Heath from Keele University.

Geoffrey Heath has been a fellow in Public Sector Accounting at Keele University since August 2010, having previously been a lecturer in accounting there. He came to Keele in September 2002 from Staffordshire University where he was an academic for many years. Before that he worked in NHS finance, qualifying as a chartered management accountant. He has a degree in Politics and Sociology from the University of Kent and a PGCE from Liverpool University. His research interests concern resource allocation and management, performance evaluation and accountability in the public sector. He has been engaged for some time in collaborative research and evaluation in health, social care, community safety, urban renewal and localism. Since retiring from lecturing, he has been involved as a practitioner on financial inclusion projects.

Chapter 7
Leadership and System Thinking in the Modern Ambulance Service

Andy Newton and Graham Harris

Introduction

Many definitions of leadership turn, entirely understandably, on the ability to motivate individuals to higher levels of performance, such as the quote from Peter Drucker below which extols:

> ...Leadership is lifting a person's vision to higher sights, the raising of a person's performance to a higher standard, the building of a personality beyond its normal limitations. (Peter Drucker (1909–2005))

Nevertheless, no amount of motivational zeal, leadership frameworks or entreaties for improvements in leadership generally is likely to succeed unless the relationship between the leader and the system and procedures with which they work is fully considered. Peter Scholtes (1998) in his book *the Leader's Handbook: Making Things Happen: Getting Things Done*, amongst others, recognises this fact, and organisations such as the military and others emphasise the relationship between doctrine, organisation, culture and leadership at every level. The issue for ambulance service leaders and for paramedics is that the systems within which they operate are often poorly understood, underdeveloped and increasingly in something of a state of flux. As the demands for service grow, finances contract or at least do not keep pace, and the role of the paramedic, who are rapidly morphing into one of a mobile healthcare provider, continues to expand.

A. Newton (✉)
South East Coast Ambulance Service, Surrey Office, The Horseshoe,
SM7 2AS Banstead, Surrey, UK
e-mail: Andy.Newton@secamb.nhs.uk

G. Harris
College of Paramedics, The Exchange, Express Park, TA6 4RR Bridgwater, UK

© Springer International Publishing Switzerland 2015
P. Wankhade, K. Mackway-Jones (eds.), *Ambulance Services,*
DOI 10.1007/978-3-319-18642-9_7

Effective leadership is, therefore, unlikely if there is a lack of clarity regarding the organisation's role or the systems and process that collectively make up the system itself. What, for example, is the organisation's doctrine? Essentially, the principles and beliefs that underpin the reason for the service's existence, for example, is it fundamentally a transport organisation or a provider of mobile health care? Every decision in respect of finances, the education and training of paramedics, equipment, vehicles and all importantly the 'concept of operation' and flow is dependent upon answering this question.

The transition from a traditional health transport role is therefore hampered, as are any associated reforms and modernisation effort, by a lack of clarity in these areas and also has widespread implications for the workforce. The situation in much of the UK ambulance service today is also exacerbated by the differing cultures within management, itself, partly negatively influenced by the above and the constant requirements to meet sometimes clinically questionable, but rigorously imposed, national targets, often relating to response times (Wankhade 2011, 2012). These damaging effects in terms of the retardation of professionalisation of paramedics, themselves, have been discussed in 'Still Blue-Collar after all these Years?'(McCann et al. 2013). There is, indeed, a high price to pay in terms of delays in releasing the full potential of paramedics in such circumstances. This chapter discusses the context in which ambulance service leaders have to operate and will set out some of the system changes that might help counteract the many current challenges to leadership at all levels of the ambulance service and to paramedics working at every level of the Paramedic Post Registration Career Framework, College of Paramedics (2015).

A Challenging Leadership Environment

A few decades ago, ambulance personnel were regarded as essentially manual labourers, employed primarily as 'drivers', with first-aid training courses provided by the voluntary aid societies, principally the St John Ambulance Brigade. The task assigned to ambulance crews was a relatively simple one; the service itself was generally regarded as something of a *Cinderella service* in comparison to the other more established emergency services.

Vehicles, equipment and training were rudimentary, and, while science had developed, modern resuscitation techniques (Safar et al. 1958; Kouwenhoven et al. 1960) had yet to be widely adopted. The technologies taken for granted today (automated external defibrillators (AEDs), 12 lead ECG machines, etc.) were the weight of a small family car often requiring mains power to operate. Only in the late 1960s, with the publication of two major national reports (Ministry of Health, Scottish Home and Health Department 1966, 1967) did the situation begin to change. These reports followed an earlier BBC panorama broadcast (British Broadcasting Corporation, BBC 1963), which identified major weaknesses in the ambulance service.

The dominant philosophy in the 1960s, still echoed in the media today, is that the ambulance service exists to serve the needs of the seriously ill and injured and to transport patients to local hospitals, a concept that can be traced to a much earlier period of pre-hospital care. Dominique Jean Larrey, a French surgeon of the Napoleonic period, is often credited as the originator of the 'modern' ambulance and the developer of triage. In many ways, he is the father of ambulance services (Richardson 2000).

Larrey's rigorous focus in developing the life-saving potential of early pre-hospital treatments has become a guiding principle and has shaped the concept of the operation of ambulance services since. Indeed, the service's reputation accelerated dramatically in the 1970s and 1980s, precisely because it became far more capable at saving lives (and managing serious cardiac illness, in particular). This was largely due to the work of pioneers such as Douglas Chamberlain and Peter Baskett, who developed paramedic advanced resuscitation services with a particular focus on cardiac care in the UK (Chamberlain et al. 1976; Baskett et al. 1976). Today's world is a radically different place, and the pattern of epidemiological demand has changed significantly. Yet, Larrey's inspiring and beguiling principles continue to exercise a strong influence over the culture, ethos and role of paramedics and doctors, who shape the ambulance service and influence other development such as the new sub-speciality of pre-hospital emergency medicine.

This is probably the wrong paradigm for ambulance. services in the modern world and may be leading ambulance services in the wrong direction or at least distorting public and professional perceptions, thereby limiting the speed at which the service and paramedic practice adapts to the needs of most patients today. Larrey's work helped inform the subsequent development of the Union Army's medical services during the American Civil War with his ideas being translated into the civilian setting in a number of American cities after the war (Post and Treiber 2002). A visiting Liverpool surgeon, Reginald Harrison, was so impressed by what he saw of the ambulance services in America in 1881, that he introduced a similar service in England on his return, setting the pattern in the UK and elsewhere (Burr 1969).

The model worked well during the industrial age and adapted to the modern plagues of the twentieth century with what the European Resuscitation Council called the 'first hour quintet of cardiac arrest, chest pain, stroke, acute breathlessness and major trauma'. But these, and other life-threatening conditions, no longer represent the core demand for most ambulance services. This is gradually being recognised in the UK (Martin and Swinburn 2012) and abroad, the acuity of patients does appear to be changing as a recent study shows (Munjal et al. 2012). Nevertheless, emergency ambulance providers have been slow to react and appear to struggle with defining what 'appropriate' emergency ambulance care actually is (Judge 2004).

In the twenty-first century, life-saving remains a key objective and a key competency for paramedics and ambulance services delivering ever more effective services for patients with life-threatening conditions, recently acknowledged in a position statement from the National Emergency Medical Service (EMS) Advisory Council (National EMS Advisory Council 2009). However, it can no longer be regarded as other than one priority amongst many responsibilities as recently acknowledged by a leading EMS commentator, who lamented the slow response of American services to recognise a need for change (Heightman and McCallion 2011). What is required today is a new guiding principle coupled with a new concept of operation taking into account demographic change, a professionalised paramedic workforce and harsh realities of the current economic climate.

Though the modern ambulance service has demonstrated greatly enhanced clinical capabilities in a short period, transport continues to be the dominant theme, and new concepts of operation, based on a more clinical, decision-focused approach have not yet become fully embedded, resulting in a delay of progress.

Ambulance Services and the Need to 'Shift Left'

The challenges of the economic climate will continue for some time, therefore, ambulance services need to absorb increased activity (much of it comprising what, in earlier years, would have been dealt with by primary care) and assimilate this into a lower unit cost, all against a backdrop of falling funding. Indeed, 999 call volumes have increased from approximately 1 million in 1966 to over 8 million today, with a massive increase in the order of 100 % occurring between 1996 (3.2 million) and the 8.47 million calls received during 2013–2014 (Health and Social Care Information Centre 2014), with a continuing upward trend today, albeit with a reduced growth.

As far back as 1999, informed commentators were describing the trend as 'astonishing' (Carney 1999), while others opined about the legitimacy of demand and 'inappropriate' use (Palazzo et al. 1998). Such concerns are not new; in 1903 (Hadfield 1903), the Liverpool horse-drawn ambulance service was observed and received the following comment:

> …there can be little doubt in the mind of an independent observer that a considerable proportion of those carried in ambulances get there, either directly or indirectly through the abuse of drink. Either their own bad habits have been the cause of injury, or they have been the victims of the drunken violence of others. (Municipal Ambulance Work. The Windsor Magazine (1903))

He also noted that there were a small number of 'chronic malingerers', who were encountered during his forays while observing ambulance crews. Papers regarding 'inappropriate' use seem less common today, perhaps due to the introduction of triage systems from 1996 (NHS Management Executive 1996), but more likely due to studies showing that many of these cases are generated by genuine concerns over the severity of systems (Sanders 2000), due to patients finding that accessing care, particularly out of hours (Lakhani et al. 2007), was 'confusing' or because of the actions of bystanders whose public spiritedness it would be churlish to deride (Volans 1998). It could also be partly as a result of the failure of media campaigns to mitigate the issue and perhaps also because the advent of tariff creates an incentive to deal with demand that presents itself. After a review of the literature (Snooks et al 1998), it was suggested that ambulance services should worry less about 'appropriateness' and devote more effort to providing appropriate care.

Raising productivity and ensuring high standards of clinical service are essential, but is no longer a sufficiently expansive objective for paramedics or the ambulance

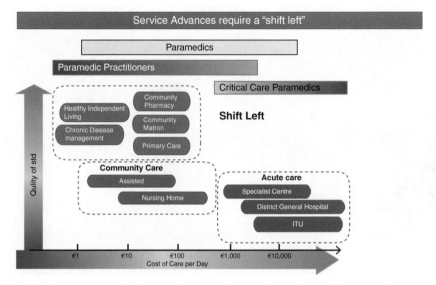

Fig. 7.1 Diagram demonstrating how the role of paramedics and specialist paramedics can be 'shifted left'. *ITU* Intensive Treatment Unit (Adapted from Rasmus 2009)

service. Further urgent reforms in operation and the introduction of modern managerial methods are now essential. The current model as it stands will continue to transport many patients to hospitals unnecessarily, which is unsatisfactory and unsustainable when other options are available.

There are several keys to accelerating and completing the changes that are urgently needed. The first is to recognise that a major shift in health care is taking place within the developed world, but it is less explicit than might be expected and not yet fully entrenched in policy. This change is mostly financially driven, but clinical benefits also exist, if executed effectively. This movement of patients from high-acuity and high-cost areas on the right side of Fig. 7.1, to less costly locations on the left, illustrates this phenomenon. The diagram also shows that in this example, ambulance services can specialise or tier their staff with, for example, paramedics developed in primary, urgent care, while others are focused on critical care. The model also promotes the move to undergraduate status of student paramedics.

Transforming Ambulance Services Before It Is Too Late

The second challenge has been recognised for some time and was the subject of a detailed study *Life in the Fast Lane*, published by the Audit Commission (1998), and considered again in 2011 in the National Audit Office's report *Transforming Ambulance Services* (National Audit Office (NAO) 2011) and relates to efficiency and the application of lean methods.

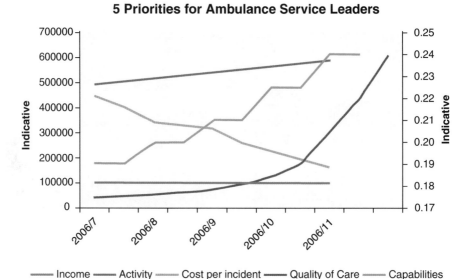

Fig. 7.2 'Spinning plates': Five priorities for ambulance service leaders

Both reports skirted the issues of what real transformation in terms of the concept of operation might look like, but they did make useful observations and suggestions as to how greater productivity could be encouraged in the ambulance section. In some respects, these findings paralleled earlier American ambulance reports which set out the primary goals that all emergency ambulance services should strive for response time reliability, clinical sophistication, customer satisfaction and economic efficiency (Stout 1983a, b; American Ambulance Association 2008).

These principles would fall into what are often termed 'lean' management methods and derived from Deming's quality management theories (Ryan 2002). The previous American reports(Stout 1983a; Stout 1983b) demonstrate a useful metric, termed 'unit hour utilisation', to determine the productivity of an ambulance service by simply dividing the number of patients transported, or patient contacts, by the availability of ambulance time expressed in hours. For example, an ambulance service producing four unit hours of ambulance time, and moving one patient would be operating at a 0.25 level of utilisation/productivity.

This simple system has yet to be widely adopted in the UK, although discussion regarding a standardised approach is now underway. However, a continuing quest for higher productivity and stronger response time performance will no longer be sufficient as the following points will illustrate.

The diagram in Fig. 7.2 brings together the external forces and some countermeasures with the red line showing rising demand and the lower, *blue line* reflecting falling income. Bringing down the unit cost is therefore imperative through enhanced utilisation (or improved productivity), shown in *green*.

To address the current pressures caused by increasing low-acuity demand, the key strategic priority should be to recoup and reinvest a proportion of the funds derived from enhanced utilisation to develop new clinical capabilities (income), while ensuring that conventional indicators of quality (activity), such as response time performance, patient safety, clinical governance and patient experience continually improve as well.

In this context, improved capabilities revolve around developing specialist paramedic practice to address patient needs in both primary and critical care as the primary means of making the system generate the productivity gains. Delivery of primary care would include the assessment and treatment of a wide range of clinical presentations such as wound management, near patient testing and a wide range of referral options. Critical care would include patient assessment, the provision of a broader range of therapeutics, advanced airway management, cardiovascular support and the introduction of new technologies such as ultrasound, to help guide treatment in the field, ideally, with the provision of online support from more senior paramedics and medical staff where necessary.

The conundrum for the ambulance services and the paramedic profession is how to continue to add value and improve quality in a financially constrained environment. Some might be tempted to reduce (or at least not to improve) clinical quality or to settle for more traditional transport-oriented concepts of operation. This approach fails to grasp the opportunities associated with the use of more highly qualified paramedics, such as specialist and advanced paramedics, which would unlock the prospect of delivering mobile health care and adopting a gate-keeping function. Such approaches are predicated on the basis that unnecessary transportation to hospital can have adverse financial consequences for the rest of the health economy and only works if the issues considered are at the 'whole healthcare system' level, rather than considering the ambulance service to be one of many silos.

If the choice is to continue with the predominant transport model, it is possible, although by no means certain, that private ambulance providers might be able to accomplish this more cheaply than many existing National Health Services (NHS) ambulance services. However, this might be achieved at the expense of transmitting larger numbers of patients into overburdened emergency departments, unless the private services invested in the same work force capabilities are as advocated above. An opportunity to develop an integrated, system-wide approach could also be lost resulting in increased cost and clinical risk as large numbers of patients are unnecessarily taken to hospital, ramping up downstream costs.

Clinical care came under the microscope at the turn of the century, with an ambulance service association sponsored paper (Nicholl et al. 1999). This may have helped influence the 2001 Department of Health's glimmering of interest in widening the ambulance service's role in reforming emergency care (DH 2001), spawning a veritable industry of 'reforming' publications. These went largely unchallenged from the ambulance service, but for the occasional, cautionary note from commentators, who questioned the scale and wisdom of the proposed changes in respect of the ambulance service (Judge 2004). By 2005, the report *Taking Health Care to the Patient* (DH 2005) condensed these policy ideas and other initiatives into a document focused specifically on the ambulance service role.

The report made the correct diagnosis but the implementation of the necessary changes was, arguably, poorly executed. The second edition of the report (Association of Ambulance Chief Executives 2011), was the closest the NHS ambulance services have had to current policy, but while some of the recommendations have seen some action, the failure to build them into the NHS operating framework, and the lack of clear doctrine has attenuated the report's effect. This situation has improved with the publication of the urgent and emergency care review (NHS England 2013), which brings together many of the necessary ingredients for positive change in the NHS. Notably, it also recognises and supports the need for a change of paradigm from transport to treatment at the point of contact for the ambulance service and paramedics, placing this in the context of systematic organisational changes designed to move the focus from hospitals to a reformed and reinforced set of community services.

A Changing NHS Model

The NHS today is strikingly similar to that which was established at its inception in 1948 (NHS 2014), a surprising finding, given the very dramatic changes in demography, disease patterns (epidemiology), social norms, medical technology, increased medical specialisation and other factors. There is still a large reliance upon acute hospitals, typically district general hospitals (DGHs) which, until quite recently, were generally regarded as capable of dealing with the majority of ill health and injury from catchment populations that do not generally exceed 250,000 people. In reality, hospitals provide only 10 % of the health care for their communities, with the other 90 % being provided by the primary care services, but the dependency of patients who are admitted to hospitals is increasing.

In the future, it is likely that hospitals will be graded into specialist emergency centres and urgent care centres, with the former serving a larger population base of approximately 1,000,000 or possibly larger, the exact size is still somewhat uncertain. There will be a continuing emphasis upon services provided in the community, with a concomitant need for higher levels of interservice integration than has been achieved before. Such arrangements, particularly in terms of the role of grading hospitals, although less so in the provision of supporting community services, have been common in North America, while many European and other industrialised countries have achieved both changes in hospital roles and more reliance upon community services decades ago. The specialist emergency centres in particular are expected to provide more sophisticated services for those patients requiring cardiology, neurological care, major vascular surgery, complex trauma care and intensive therapy services. There will be many occasions when it will be in the direct interest of patients to be directly transported to such facilities, especially so when one considers the acutely time-dependent nature of many medical and surgical emergencies, such as heart attack, stroke and major haemorrhage.

It is increasingly apparent that at least some ambulance services in the UK are developing, almost by default, a doctrine of mobile healthcare provision, hospital and admission avoidance and becoming increasingly integrated into the wider NHS. The emergency function remains, but the resultant cultures and operating methods

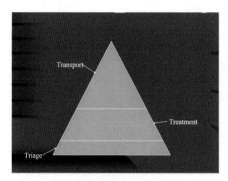 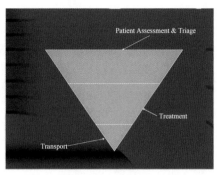

Fig. 7.3 The changing concept of operation of the ambulance service

to achieve both effective emergency response and meeting undifferentiated urgent care needs are different and not always easily reconciled. Supporting this new reality requires a change in clinical concept of operations (CONOPS) which literally turns historical operating models on 'their head', generating a new set of systems and processes (see Fig. 7.3). Virtually all strategic and tactical decisions that managers and leaders make, whether in respect of the training and education of staff, equipment, vehicles, the employment of triage systems and clinical governance arrangements, these decisions are invariably dependent upon both the doctrine and the resulting concept of operation. If unclear as to which model is appropriate in a given area, the result is likely to be a lack of clarity by the wider organisation, leaders, staff and potentially patients too. Such a situation risks compromise and provides a poor basis for achieving a high-quality result for patients.

The clinical ramifications of these changes are substantial, both operationally and in regard to professional issues for paramedics, upon whom the preponderance of the new responsibilities fall. In reality, this evolution in role has been led by patient demand and reconfiguration within the wider NHS, particularly those that have affected general practice, including the amendments in the contractual obligations of general practitioners (GPs). As previously discussed, the 999 call volumes have increased, with 100 % occurring during the past two decades. Essentially, the report 'Taking Health Care to the Patient'(DH 2005), has made a virtue out of necessity and recommended that the ambulance service take on the responsibilities of a mobile healthcare provider, with the broad objective of reducing the number of patient transports to hospital by approximately 25 % or roughly 1.5 million journeys per annum. The more recent review report on urgent and emergency care (NHS England 2013), adopts a strategic reappraisal of the wider NHS context and provides a considered framework for meaningful change.

The operational model for delivering ambulance services will need to be radically revised and this will need to be accomplished at the same time as incorporating the many professional and educational changes that will need to accompany the process. The model will have many differences to the transport-based operations provided today. It will be 'front loaded', in the sense that the ambulance clinicians attending patients will increasingly be paramedics with further skills in patient assessment, management and referral. For these staff to be effective, it will be important to have a range of referral opportunities, therapies, good communications and procedures with the local health economy, as well as good relations, particularly with GPs, some of whom will be responsible for much of the clinical training and support of staff.

This modernisation effort is far-reaching and involves a large number of stakeholders and will need to complete the efficiency recommendations identified and discussed throughout the chapter. The potential benefits of achieving and implementing this within ambulance services has already been realised (Health Education England 2014; Francis 2013). To achieve these aspirations requires a clear business and quality performance framework for the twenty-first century patient care that represents a logical approach and context for the leaders of tomorrow's ambulance service leaders.

Conclusion

Effective leadership can only take place in the context of 'systems thinking' coupled with the other well-established leadership competencies. But effective system thinking itself relies upon having a clear doctrine, describing what the ambulance services role actually is and delivering mobile health care in an integrated manner. The doctrine must be coupled with a clear CONOPS which is likely to see the traditional transport function progressively replaced by a more skilled and educated paramedic profession, capable of delivering critical decision-making, managing and treating increasing numbers of patients presenting with urgent, primary care and emergency conditions, thus making the paramedic more relevant to present and future patient populations. Future clinical leaders will be able to discharge their responsibilities and articulate a shared, attractive vision all the more convincingly when the relationship between generic leadership skills and a well-conceived system design are transparent and understood by all.

References

American Ambulance Association. (2008). *Structured for quality: Best practices in designing, managing and contracting for emergency ambulance service*. McLean: American Ambulance Association.

Association of Ambulance Chief Executives. (2011). *Taking healthcare to the patient 2: A review of 6 years' progress and recommendations for the future*. London: Association of Ambulance Chief Executives.

Audit Commission. (1998). *Life in the fast lane, A: Value for money in emergency ambulance services*. London: Audit Commission Report.

Baskett, P. J., Diamond, A. W., & Cochrane, D. F. (1976). Urban mobile resuscitation training and service. *British Journal of Anaesthesia, 48*(4), 377–385.

British Broadcasting Corporation (BBC). (1963). Panorama. The ambulance services are under fire. http://www.bbc.co.uk/archive/nhs/5161.shtml. Accessed 16 Aug 2014.

Burr, M. L. (1969). A concise history of ambulance services in Britain. *The Medical Officer, 121,* 228–235 (Reprinted in Ambulance UK 2001, 16, 161–181).

Carney, C. J. (1999). Prehospital care—a UK perspective. *British Medical Bulletin, 55*(4), 757–766.

Chamberlain, D. A., Brown, P. M., & Briggs, R. S. (1976). The Brighton resuscitation ambulances: A continuing experiment in prehospital care by ambulance staff. *British Medical Journal, 2,* 1161–1165.

College of Paramedics. (2015). *Paramedic Post Registration—Career Framework* (3rd ed.). Bridgwater: College of Paramedics.

Department of Health (DH). (2001). *Reforming emergency care: First steps to a new approach.* London: Department of Health Publications.

Department of Health (DH). (2005). *Taking healthcare to the patient: Transforming NHS ambulance services.* London: Department of Health Publications.

Francis, R. (2013). *Mid Staffordshire NHS foundation trust public inquiry. Final report.* London: The Stationery Office.

Hadfield, H. (1903). Municipal ambulance work. *The Windsor Magazine, 18*(3), 339–437.

Heightman, A. J., & McCallion, T. (2011). Management lessons from Pinnacle: Key messages given to EMS leaders at the 2011 conference. *Journal of Emergency Medical Services, 36*(10), 50–54.

Health and Social Care Information Centre. (2014). Ambulance services, England—2013–2014 (NS). http://www.hscic.gov.uk/catalogue/PUB14601. Accessed 3 Aug 2014.

Health Education England. (2014). *Framework 15: Health education England strategic framework 2014–2029.* London: Health Education England.

Judge, T. P. (2004). "Reforming Emergency Care" and ambulance services. *Emergency Medicine Journal, 21*(2), 4.

Kouwenhoven, W. B., Jude, J. R., & Knickerbocker G. G. (1960). Closed-chest cardiac massage. *Journal of American Medical Association, 173,* 1064–1067.

Lakhani, M., Fernandes, A., & Archard, D. (2007). *Urgent care: A position statement from the royal college of general practitioners.* London: The Royal College of General Practitioners.

Martin, J., & Swinburn, A. (2012). Paramedic clinical leadership. *Journal of Paramedic Practice, 4*(3), 181–182.

McCann, J., Granter, E., Hyde, P., & Hassard, J. (2013). Still blue-collar after all these years? An ethnography of the professionalization of emergency ambulance work. *Journal of Management Studies, 50*(5), 750–776.

Ministry of Health, Scottish Home and Health Department. (1966) *Report by the working party on ambulance training and equipment: Part 1—training.* London: HMSO.

Ministry of Health, Scottish Home and Health Department. (1967). *Report by the working party on ambulance training and equipment: Part 2—equipment.* London: HMSO.

Munjal, K. G., Silverman, R. A., Freese, J., Braun, J. D., Bradley, J. K., Kaufman, B., et al. (2011). Utilization of emergency medical services in a large urban area: Description of call types and temporal trends. *Pre-Hospital Emergency Care, 15*(3), 371–380.

National Audit Office (NAO). (2011). *Transforming NHS ambulance services. Report by the comptroller and auditor general. HC 1086 Session 2010–2012.* London: The Stationery Office.

National Health Service (NHS). (2014). The history of the NHS in England. http://www.nhs.uk/NHSEngland/thenhs/nhshistory/Pages/the-nhs%20history.aspx. Accessed 17 Aug 2014.

National EMS Advisory Council. (2009). EMS makes a difference: Improving clinical outcomes and downstream healthcare savings. A Position Statement of the National EMS Advisory Council. www.ems.gov/pdf/nemsac-dec2009.pdf. Accessed 16 Aug 2014.

National Health Service Management Executive. (1996). *Review of ambulance performance standards: Final report of the Steering Committee.* London: NHS Executive.

Nicholl, J., Turner, J., & Martin, D. (1999). *The future of ambulance services in the United Kingdom: A strategic review of options for the future of ambulance services carried out on behalf of the ambulance service association: Towards perfect vision 2000–2010.* London: Ambulance Service Association.

NHS England. (2013). *High quality care for all, now and for future generations: Transforming urgent and emergency care services in England—urgent and emergency care review end of phase 1 report*. Leeds: Urgent and Emergency Care Review Team.

Palazzo, F. F., Warner, O. J., Harron, M., & Morrison, W. R. (1998). Misuse of the London ambulance service: How much and why? *Journal of Accident and Emergency Medicine. 15*(6), 368–370.

Post, C., & Treiber, M. (2002). History. In: A. E. Kuehl (Ed.), *Prehospital systems and medical oversight* (3rd ed.). Dubuque: Kendall/Hunt Publishing Company.

Rasmus, W. (2009). *Listening to the future, why it's everybody's business: Microsoft executive leadership series*. New Jersey: Wiley.

Richardson, R. (2000). *Larrey: Surgeon to Napoleon's imperial guard (revised ed.)*. London: Quiller Press.

Ryan, J. L. (2002). Quality management. In: A. E. Kuehl (Ed.), *Prehospital systems and medical oversight* (3rd ed.). Dubuque: Kendall/Hunt Publishing Company.

Safar, P., Lourdes, A., Escarraga, M. D., & Elam, O. J. (1958). A comparison of mouth-to-mouth and mouth-to-airway methods of artificial respiration with chest pressure arm lift methods. *New England Journal of Medicine, 258*(14), 671–677.

Sanders, J. (2000). A review of health professional attitudes and patient perceptions on 'inappropriate' accident and emergency attendances—The implications for current minor injury service provision in England and Wales. *Journal of Advanced Nursing, 31*(5), 1097–1105.

Scholtes, P. R. (1998). *The leader's handbook: Making things happen: Getting things done*. New York: McGraw-Hill.

Snooks, H., Wrigley, H., George, S., Thomas, E., Smith, H., & Glasper, A. (1998). Appropriateness of use of emergency ambulances. *Journal of Accident and Emergency Medicine, 15*(4), 212–215.

Stout, J.L. (1983a). Measuring your system. *Journal of Emergency Medical Services, 8*(1), 884–891.

Stout, J. L. (1983b). System status management: The strategy for ambulance placement. *Journal of Emergency Medical Services, 8*(5), 22–32.

Volans, A. (1998). Use and abuse of the ambulance service. *Pre-Hospital Immediate Care, 2,* 190–192.

Wankhade, P. (2011). Performance measurement and the UK emergency ambulance service: Unintended consequences of the ambulance response time targets. *International Journal of Public Sector Management, 24*(5), 384–402.

Wankhade, P. (2012). Different cultures of management and their relationships with organizational performance: Evidence from the UK ambulance service. *Public Money & Management, 32*(5), 381–388.

Prof. Andy Newton QAM, FCPara, BSC (Hons), MSc, PhD is a consultant paramedic and director of Clinical Operations, South East Coast Ambulance Service NHS Foundation Trust (SECAMB) since July 2006. He is also the current chair of the College of Paramedics, the Professional Body for Paramedics in the UK. His executive role was coupled with the first appointment of a Consultant Paramedic in the UK, which covered the key areas of clinical practice, professional leadership, teaching, service modernisation and research. He is currently responsible for the Clinical Operations Directorate involving 2500 operational and control room personnel, professional standards and the innovation, research and service improvement priorities within the Trust budget of £108 million. Formerly clinical director for Sussex Ambulance Service NHS Trust, Andy has extensive experience in the NHS ambulance service and education sector, in clinical, educational, managerial and senior leadership roles. He is a visiting professor at Edge Hill University and the University of Surrey. He is also the current chair of the College of Paramedic and partner and visitor for the Health & Care Professions Council (HCPC).

Graham Harris MSc, BSc, PGCE, Chartered MCIPD, FCPara is the director of Professional Standards at the College of Paramedics, UK. Graham has a long and credible career as a paramedic, acquired over a period of 44 years in the military, NHS and Higher Education areas of paramedic practice, within the clinical, managerial, education and research aspect. Graham is committed to supporting the ongoing development of the paramedic profession. He has authored several publications and articles, and is the successful co-editor of Assessment Skills for Paramedics, and the acclaimed, Clinical Leadership for Paramedics. In his role as the College of Paramedics Director of Professional Standards, he has been instrumental in the application for paramedics to obtain NHS bursaries, the synthesis and publication of the Paramedic Curriculum Guidance 3rd edition, and the Paramedic Post Registration Career Framework, and the Paramedic Post Registration Clinical Competence Framework. His vision is to see the College of Paramedics achieve the Royal College of Paramedics status.

Chapter 8
Ambulance Service Modernisation

Robert Till and Anthony Marsh

Introduction and Background

A significant proportion of work the modern ambulance service undertakes involves the treatment of patients at the scene of an accident or illness and if necessary the conveyance, where appropriate of the patient, to the nearest appropriate acute facility able to deal with the patient's condition. However, an increasing proportion of work involves the stabilisation of patients, delivery of more advanced treatment and complex decision-making based on comprehensive patient assessment. Ambulance services engage fully with acute and community health professionals, working alongside them to ensure rapid and effective treatment of patients in the most challenging and life-threatening situations.

In addition to modernising clinical practice, ambulance services have to reassess and modernise their finances. The King's Fund and Institute for Fiscal Studies (Appleby et al. 2010) have estimated that, with near static real-term increases in funding, the National Health Services (NHS) will have to get 4–6% more for its money year on year to do little more than maintain existing standards of care (in the face of inflation and rising demand). In 2012, Andrew Lansley, the then secretary of state for health, reaffirmed the previous government's commitment to making efficiency savings totalling £ 20 billion by 2014. Quality, innovation, productivity and prevention (QIPP) is a large-scale transformational programme for the NHS,

R. Till (✉)
West Midlands Ambulance Service NHS FT, Trust HQ, Waterfront Business Park,
Waterfront Way, DY5 1LX Brierley Hill, West Midlands, UK
e-mail: Robert.Till@wmas.nhs.uk

A. Marsh
West Midlands Ambulance Service NHS FT, Executive Office, Trust HQ, Waterfront Business
Park, Waterfront Way, DY5 1LX Brierley Hill, West Midlands, UK
e-mail: Anthony.Marsh@wmas.nhs.uk

© Springer International Publishing Switzerland 2015   95
P. Wankhade, K. Mackway-Jones (eds.), *Ambulance Services,*
DOI 10.1007/978-3-319-18642-9_8

involving all NHS staff, clinicians, patients and the voluntary sector. It will improve the quality of care the NHS delivers whilst making up to £ 20 billion of efficiency savings by 2014–2015, which will be reinvested in frontline care.

At the end of 2012, the Office of National Statistics (ONS) confirmed that Britain's economic growth was broadly flat (Hardie et al. 2013). Ambulance services therefore need to ensure that they find and optimise resources, organisational knowledge and talent. Ambulance services needed to meet the impact of recession and efficient services also needed to be quality services; therefore, effective leadership is critical.

In January 2013, NHS medical director, Professor Sir Bruce Keogh, announced a comprehensive review of the NHS urgent and emergency care system in England (NHS England 2013). The report released in November 2013 acknowledged that the current pressures on ambulance trusts are unsustainable. The ambulance service is still seen as the safety net for patients and increasingly picks up the patients who fall through the net of inadequate urgent and social care. The ambulance service is being asked to develop into the mobile treatment service desired by Keogh but must secure investment to allow the development and transformation into this new role. The ambulance service of the future has an enormous role to play in helping save the NHS money. Ambulance services have already started this process by working in collaboration with urgent care providers or providing 111 services, for example.

Organisational Development

An organisational development department plays a crucial role in developing a modern ambulance service. The success of a service rests on its leaders and staff. In order to be successful, an ambulance service must address skill deficits and build talent in order to future-proof it. This success can be measured in several ways, including improved quality of patient care, improved clinical outcomes and improved staff satisfaction surveys.

In the face of continuous change, an ambulance trust has to be flexible, offer employee and patient satisfaction, incremental development, and it should have the ability to attract and retain talent and strengthened ability to meet challenging new targets. Continuous change, is a given, in any progressive organisation that wishes to adapt to meet emerging needs. Appointed and current leaders need to have the strength and courage to lead innovative change that inspires and motivates staff to adopt new ways of working.

Key appointments within a trust need to focus on encouraging applications from leaders who can support the continuing development of the environment and conditions for transformational change that reward creativity and innovation. Ambulance trusts need to foster, nurture, recruit, train and retain staff at all levels. Staff need to be encouraged and empowered to exercise leadership with increasing confidence. The national QIPP agenda clearly summarises the challenges NHS leaders face. To achieve this, staff must be empowered to come up with the right ideas, and they must have the knowledge, skill and will to meet quality standards.

A key finding in the independent inquiry into Mid Staffordshire NHS Foundation Trust (Francis 2013) was that organisational culture is the key to providing good care for patients by providing a supportive working environment for staff:

> If there is one lesson to be learnt, I suggest it is that the people must always come before numbers. It is the individual experiences that lie behind statistics and benchmarks and action plans that really matter, and that is what must never be forgotten when policies are being made and implemented. (Robert Francis QC)

Understanding the organisations' culture is a vital part of the strategic process as it allows us to become aware of our perceptions, influence the way we process and interpret our experience, both as individuals and members of an organisation. Ambulance services must, through a whole system approach, seek organisational change defined as new patterns of action, belief and attitudes amongst staff.

In order to be effective, it is imperative that there is a whole system approach. This approach will ensure that any programmes, interventions or processes are aligned to a trusts vision, values and strategic goals. The focus will be on a joined-up plan which is fair, equitable, inclusive and transparent and which drives the desired organisational culture.

One of the key priorities an ambulance service has to consider is their workforce. We have highlighted some of the key elements next.

Workforce Planning

Having the right roles populated by people with the right knowledge, skills and attitudes is vital to organisational success. Ambulance services are presented with many challenges including varying physical environments, patient demographics and ways of working (born from historical services).

Workforce planning needs to be strategically positioned and informed by and aligned to the Trusts Integrated Business Plan (IBP). The process involves forecasting, on a 5-year rolling basis, area by area, likely presenting conditions and emergencies of patients and the roles, competencies and skills needed to respond effectively. This forecasted plan will inform the organisational learning needs analysis and plan to ensure that we have the capability and capacity to respond.

Succession Planning

Succession planning can be broadly defined as identifying future potential leaders to fill key positions. Once key roles and competencies have been identified through workforce planning, there needs to be an effective process through personal development reviews (PDRs), team and personal development plans (PDPs) and effective knowledge management, to ensure the right people are in the right posts.

To ensure a continuous flow of staff, there needs to be process in place from a number of pipelines into a trust. These can include work experience, engagement with universities, schools and colleges, internal and external career events and, more recently, being a key stakeholder in a university training college.

Going forward, Health Education England (HEE) must take more responsibility for working with trusts to develop national workforce planning and ensuring that this is funded appropriately and not left to local regional ambulance trusts to fund. There is a need to ensure that existing staff are developed to take on new roles and some of this must be provided by HEE and their local education and training boards.

Filling senior roles in ambulance trusts, especially operations roles and CEO posts, is an ongoing problem and more must be done to offer development opportunities for talented staff to move into these roles in time.

Improving Clinical Care and Outcomes for Patients

Paramedics are called to attend patients with critical medical conditions or traumatic injuries as well as primary care complaints such as patients with infections, rashes and long-term care needs. Ambulance services have adapted and are introducing new systems to ensure patients get the best level of care. This is demonstrated in the next few subsections.

Critical Care

Ambulance services play a vital part in the successful treatment of patients experiencing a stroke, trauma, heart attack or cardiac arrest. In recent years, the networks for these patients have identified the most appropriate hospitals for treatment, which may not always be the closest healthcare facility. Ambulance services have had to adapt by giving frontline clinicians extra training to be able to facilitate the longer transfer times. Ambulance services may also need to consider adjusting resourcing levels in order to continue to provide quality patient care as the extra journey time to hospital impacts the amount of vehicles that are available to respond to emergencies.

Paramedics are trained to ensure that patients receive optimum clinical care and are conveyed to the most appropriate treatment centre for their presenting condition. In order to be able to care for patients during longer transfer times, paramedics have been given extra training and equipment. In trauma cases, this equipment includes extra drug therapies, intraosseous devices, dressings which contain clotting agents and pelvic splints.

Paramedics based in the ambulance control room maintain contact with crews to offer clinical advice, give support regarding the treatment of patients and advise on the most appropriate destination hospital. They are also able to put crews in contact with an experienced pre-hospital doctor who will be able to speak to them, offering advice and support 24 h a day, 365 days a year.

An example of a critical care network is the trauma network. Patients are identified as needing to attend a specialist trauma centre by the use of a 'trauma tool scoring system'. Injuries and vital signs fall into various categories which will decide which type of hospital a patient is taken. This could be a regional trauma centre, trauma unit or local hospital.

When a patient is considered to be 'trauma tool positive', the ambulance crew will contact the trauma desk in the emergency operations centre (EOC). This desk is staffed by senior paramedics who will have expert advice to offer both clinically and in regard to where the patient should be taken. As this desk coordinates trauma within the whole region, they have update information on where recent patients have been taken by other ambulance crews. This is important as not to overload the same trauma centre with multiple patients at the same time. Clinicians on scene, hospital trauma team leaders and the trauma desk are able to undertake a conference call to determine the best care for the patient.

To deliver the highest level of care to trauma patients, medical emergency response incident teams (MERIT) have been created. The team, made up of an experienced pre-hospital doctor and a critical care paramedic, are available 24 h a day. During daylight hours, the team crew an air ambulance, during the hours of darkness they will respond using a land vehicle.

Primary Care

At the other end of the spectrum, ambulance services work closely with primary care to reduce the number of patients conveyed to hospital by ambulance. Provision of a high standard of diagnostic equipment allows paramedics to assess and diagnose a number of conditions which can be treated either in the home or through the referral of a patient to a minor injury unit or walk-in centre. In some areas, community paramedic schemes are working alongside general practitioners (GPs) to devise and deliver care plans which allow patients with long-term conditions or at the end of life to remain safely within their own homes.

Ambulance services have traditionally always triaged emergency calls to enable control staff to prioritise calls. This triage is now developing and in order to provide the most appropriate care for the patients an ambulance response is not always required.

Trained call assessors use a medical triage system to categorise a call. The highest priority of call will require the ambulance service to arrive on scene within 8 min 75 % of the time. If the triage highlights the patient does not require an ambulance response, then alternate pathways of care will be suggested. The patient may be asked to contact their GP within 24 h or perhaps make their own way to an emergency department.

In some cases, the patient may be put through to or called back by a paramedic or nurse to further assess their needs. This clinical input may lead to an ambulance being sent to the patient, but within a given timeframe rather than immediately with the use of blue lights and sirens.

This system has now been adopted by the 111 service of which some ambulance services are the provider. 111 is a service which identifies and puts patients in contact with the most appropriate care for their needs. Using the triage system, patients will be signposted to local healthcare providers such as out-of-hours services, dentists, community care and, in the event of an emergency, the 111 service will automatically create and send an emergency call directly into the ambulance services dispatch system ensuring there is no delay.

Paramedic Education and Development

In recent years, paramedic education has moved into higher education with foundation degree-level qualifications, structured and intensive post-qualification training and continued professional development. Providing paramedics with such high levels of training will undoubtedly assist in ambulance services continuing to provide the best clinical care possible. Through the increased skills of our paramedics and better integration with primary care, ambulance crews are able to diagnose and treat more patients at the scene. Between 2009–2010 and 2012–2013, West Midlands Ambulance Service reduced the number of patients conveyed to hospital from 70% to less than 58% and anticipates reducing further to 50% by 2015 (West Midlands Ambulance Service, WMAS 2013).

The Paramedic Evidence-Based Education Project (PEEP) study conducted by the Allied Health Solutions recently (Lovegrove and Davis 2013) was carried out to develop the strategic direction of the standardisation of education and training for paramedics. It concluded that there should be a standardised approach to education and training for paramedics with a nationally agreed approach to commissioning and funding. It identified the need for paramedic students to have access to bursaries in-line with the students of other nonmedical professions. The report suggests that the academic award for paramedic preregistration should be reviewed and brought in-line with allied health professionals leading to the discontinuation of the current foundation degree. The report reviewed the current content of paramedic training and suggested knowledge and skills could be enhanced by including training in clinical leadership, end of life care, integrated care and dementia and mental health awareness. In order to carry this out, the report highlights the need for HEE and NHS England to appoint a national lead for education and training of paramedics.

Need for Information, Demand and Performance Mapping

Analysing and predicting an ambulance trusts demand and performance is essential to developing ways to improve the service to patients. Creating a specialist department consisting of business intelligence developers, informatics and operational

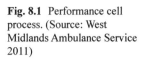

Fig. 8.1 Performance cell
process. (Source: West
Midlands Ambulance Service
2011)

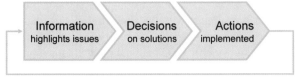

managers is one way of doing this. This department is referred to as the performance cell in this chapter.

This hybrid of skills allows for data-driven decisions to be made with the security that actions could be tested before they are fully deployed to benefit patients. It enables service delivery managers to have the confidence to move forward with plans that will deliver not only real results to the level of care for patients but also on the most efficient basis possible (Fig. 8.1).

Ambulance services have advanced information systems which collect data by time and date and can predict emergency activity with a high degree of accuracy. The sharing and use of this data is invaluable in capacity and resource planning to ensure that emergency departments are equipped to cope with demand.

The performance cell provides feature-rich information to the service delivery team to enable them to develop and refine the operational model to provide a high level of stable performance. Its aim is to help model future service developments to ensure an ambulance trust becomes a high-performing, cost-effective and stable NHS Foundation Trust. It has four key components (see Fig. 8.2):

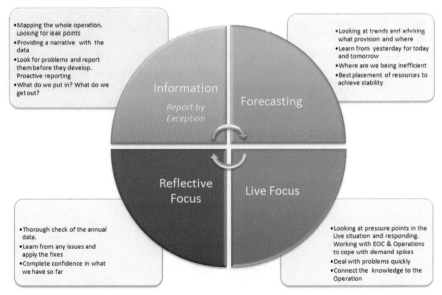

Fig. 8.2 Performance cell key components. (Source: West Midlands Ambulance Service 2011)

1. *Information*—Once the information has been produced, it is used to identify and rectify problems with the operating model that require short- to medium-term fixes. This includes issues such as reduction in lost hours, delays at hospital, efficiency metrics and national clinical indicators.
2. *Forecasting*—The performance cell produces demand profiles that allow service delivery to place on duty the correct level of resources and ensure a safe and high-performing trust. This resource plan is dynamic and takes into account seasonal variation in activity and special events.
3. *Live focus*—This information includes the live feed of activity, performance and resource information from the computer-aided dispatch system (CAD). This information is displayed on large screens to ensure visibility of key trust information that may require immediate action in the event of problems. This includes activity, resource levels, hospital delays and meal break allocation.
4. *Reflective focus*—The performance cell works closely with other departments to ensure that lessons are continually learnt and we are able to develop a high performance service. This is done through accurate ongoing analysis of the function of the trust and the development of an evidence-based decision-making model.

Outcomes of the performance cell are described below:

Results

The production of high-quality and consistent reporting and analysis measures allow for evidence-based decisions to be made that can ensure operational stability and improve performance in service delivery. The development of an accurate demand forecast for ambulance services and introduction of demand-focused rotas result in resources being on duty at times of peak activity and increased efficiency that results in a reduction in the overtime costs within a trust. Bringing together the expertise of the analysts with the data and experienced senior operational managers means an ambulance trust can react to changes in the demand profile quickly and effectively and can ensure both a safe and high-performing service are maintained.

The information and analysis processed by the performance cell has to become an intrinsic part of a services decision-making process. Any changes to an operating model should be completed following detailed analysis of the effects by the performance cell and review of the effects after the changes have been made. This change in culture will allow for significant changes to the model to be completed safely and will not risk to patient care.

Cost Effectiveness

Through the output of accurate data and forecasting intelligence, ambulance services can have the confidence in utilisation and activity modelling. This allows a more resilient response model as well as achieving a reduction in resources required through more efficient use of those available and the targeting to times of high demand. The data and reports produced have been used to identify new service delivery models and efficiencies that can be achieved safely and alongside improvements in performance. Detailed analyses and reporting of a set of key efficiency measures means that an ambulance trust is able to confidently develop its plans to ensure it can achieve the savings it requires with a 5-year plan in place. The result of these services offered by the performance cell will mean the saving achieved by other departments will be far higher than the cost of the cell and can be achieved in a safe manner.

Urgent Care: The Future

In addition to the work that is currently being undertaken, there are other opportunities for ambulance services to contribute to the improved functioning of urgent care systems. Paramedics are able to triage effectively and have the skills and training to treat a wide range of illness and injury. Several ambulance services have had success with mobile paramedic units that can be located in areas of high footfall and incidence of injury—for example a city centre on Friday and Saturday evenings. Through this experience, it is clear that paramedics could be well placed to provide minor injury and urgent care services in alternative locations alongside other health professionals.

The Keogh report (2013) proposes a fundamental shift in the provision of urgent care and advocates a system-wide transformation over the next 3–5 years, with more extensive services outside hospital and patients with more serious or life-threatening conditions receiving treatment in centres with the best clinical teams, expertise and equipment.

The report calls for the development of 999 ambulance services so that they become mobile urgent treatment services, noting that paramedics now have the skills and equipment to deliver treatments that would only have been done by doctors 10 years ago. The report also highlights that by working closely with improved community services, ambulance staff can safely manage many more patients at scene by either treating them in their own home or referring them on to other appropriate community-based services. The report adds that there are also opportunities for extending the training of paramedics to allow them to assess, prescribe for and manage patients with exacerbations of chronic illnesses, working more closely with GPs and other community health services.

Operating Model

As previously mentioned in the chapter entitled 'Dealing with Austerity', some ambulance services have chosen to completely change their operating model. This move has seen traditional ambulance stations be replaced by large central reporting hubs which facilitate crew change over, fleet maintenance, local management and training, and community ambulance stations, which is where a community paramedic is based. These can often be found in fire stations, police stations, medical establishments and shared office buildings.

This change in operating model was developed to positively improve the following:

- Improved working conditions with better facilities in each hub location
- Reduction in health and safety issues
- Improved Disability Discrimination Act 2005 compliancy

The organisation will also be a significant beneficiary (see below):

- Maximise vehicle cleanliness
- Minimise cross-infection
- Improvement in medicines management
- Maximise unit hour utilisation (UHU) through effective readiness
- Minimise unit hour (UH) wastage, whilst resources are in operation
- Maximise vehicle availability
- Minimise the critical vehicle failure rate (CVFR), fleet and equipment related
- Reduce costs by reducing the number of locations medical equipment/consumables and materials are stocked and sorted
- Ensure vehicles are only stocked to a required standard and level
- Provide assurance regarding asset control and medical equipment servicing routines
- Provide readiness arrangements for major incident assets and ensure ancillary staff exists to deploy and manage the physical assets whilst at an incident site or in training mode

This operating model works in conjunction with a system status management plan. This plan is produced by collating historical data regarding 999 calls, then by applying a formula the increased activity is accounted for. The end result is a prediction of the number of incidents which require responding to in a specified area. The plan can be fixed (areas will always present in the same priority) or dynamic (priority changes every hour). This gives staff in the control room an order to which to send vehicles to standby in priority of the predicted busiest areas. This will ensure that the time it takes to respond to life-threatening 999 calls is kept to a minimum and therefore improving clinical outcomes of patients.

By having the large central hub facilities and smaller community stations, ambulance crews do not have to be returned to a specific station and therefore the ambulances should be in the correct places to respond to 999 calls.

Located at the central hub is the 'make ready' facility which employs Ambulance Fleet Assistants (AFA). These staff are responsible for the cleaning, restocking and checking of vehicles before they are used for frontline duty. This role enables vehicles to turn around more quickly and therefore be available more quickly to respond to 999 calls. Traditionally, paramedics have had to check and stock their ambulance at the start of the shift, which can take 20–30 min. Under the 'make ready' scheme, when an ambulance crew report for duty they will have a fully stocked ambulance available to them that has been checked and can be used immediately. Likewise, if during the shift the ambulance requires restocking or cleaning because of an incident they have attended, instead of that ambulance being unavailable whilst the crew clean and restock it, the AFA will have prepared a spare ambulance, so the crew simply report back to the central hub and exchange vehicles.

Experience and Expertise in Ambulance Services

Ambulance services have developed regional, robust mechanisms for receiving calls, triaging them quickly where necessary and sending speedy responses. Call handling and response times are amongst the best in the world. With this technology and training, ambulance services are well placed to contribute more to the development of both NHS 111 and out-of-hours services, ensuring the best use of technology in the streamlining of these services.

The ambulance service is the most trusted brand in the NHS and has an excellent reputation and high satisfaction rates are expressed by our patients. The ambulance service has much more to offer in the future if commissioners can be convinced to invest in it.

Conclusion

The Association of Ambulance Chief Executives (AACE) offers an infrastructure to move forward as a sector and take a national view in a way that is perhaps unique across the NHS. They have the ability to share best practice, agree and deliver changes for the benefit of patients and the promotion of equality across all ten ambulance trusts and therefore across the country. Similarly, the way in which they work together to provide national resilience and emergency preparedness demonstrates a high level of national uniformity and resilience which could be well used to quickly implement high impact changes in the urgent and emergency care arena.

At a time of reduced public confidence in the NHS and confusion about the services that are available, ambulance services continue to be held in very high regard by the public. Patient surveys, general feedback and stakeholder engagement all show that ambulance services and paramedics as a professional group are trusted to deliver high-quality patient care and to help patients effectively navigate around the healthcare system. This position could be exploited by ensuring that ambulance services have, and are recognised to have, a central and pivotal role in agreeing and implementing improvements and developments across the spectrum of urgent and primary care, including out of hours, NHS 111 and the provision of care closer to home to avoid unnecessary hospital admissions.

References

Appleby, J., Ham, C., Imison, C., & Jennings, M. (2010). *Improving NHS productivity: More with the same not more of the same*. London: The Kings Fund.

Francis, R. (2013). *Lessons learnt and related key recommendations*. Report of the Mid Staffordshire NHS Foundation Trust Public Enquiry. Executive Summary. The Stationery Office, London, pp. 65–84.

Hardie, M., Lee, P., & Perry, F. (2013). *Impact of changes in the National Accounts and Economic Commentary for Q1 2013*. Office for National Statistics. Economic Review, June 2013.

Lovegrove, M., & Davis, J. (2013). *Maximising paramedics' contribution to the delivery of high quality and cost effective patient care*. High Wycombe: Buckinghamshire New University.

NHS England. (2013). *Transforming urgent and emergency care in England: Urgent and emergency care review, phase 1 report*. Leeds: NHS England.

West Midlands Ambulance Service. (2011). The performance cell ambulance service institute innovation award. Power Point presentation slide 2 and 4.

West Midlands Ambulance Service. (2013). Quality accounts report 2013.

Robert Till started his ambulance career in 2000. Robert has worked as a paramedic, HEMS paramedic, special operations response team responder, duty manager within the Emergency Operations Centre and Executive Officer to the CEO of West Midlands Ambulance Service. He has represented West Midlands Ambulance Service at National Events and has pursued his interest in leadership and modernising ambulance services by working closely with Dr Marsh.

Dr Anthony Marsh QAM, SBStJ, DSci (Hon), MBA, MSc, FASI started his ambulance career in Essex in 1987. He relocated as the chief executive officer of the West Midlands Ambulance Service in 2006. Anthony holds a Master of Science Degree in strategic leadership as well as a Master in Business Administration (MBA) and has been awarded a Doctorate from the University of Wolverhampton. In addition to his responsibilities as CEO he was appointed chair of the Association of Ambulance Chief Executives, lead for the National Ambulance Resilience Unit and is also the CEO of East of England Ambulance Service. Dr Marsh was awarded Queens Ambulance Service Medal in the 2014.

Chapter 9
Interoperability and Multiagency Cooperation

John Stephenson

Introduction

The ambulance service in the UK started its operations as a service provided through local government similar to the police and the fire service. As such, it was classed as a blue-light emergency service, there to respond to emergency calls from the public via the 999 emergency telephone system. The three blue-light services have developed separately as three different government departments, which have different agendas and priorities, govern them. The ambulance services are governed by the Department of Health, the Home Office governs the police forces and the fire and rescue services fall under the Department of Communities and Local Government (DCLG), therefore they have developed in different ways, with different goals for the future. On top of this, during government reorganisation during the 1970s, the ambulance service moved from the local government control to become a part of the National Health Service (NHS), and as the role of the ambulance service moved from a blue-light service to a patient transport service to a clinical care providing service, the ethos and the attitudes and behaviours of the ambulance service changed.

This historical progress has resulted in a problem with the three services that no longer naturally understand each other, and there is now a need to re-engage at both a national and local level. In the current state of financial austerity, there are financial advantages in working more closely as there can be areas where we currently duplicate activity, there are also areas where it makes more sense for a different service to take the lead.

J. Stephenson (✉)
National Ambulance Resilience Unit (NARU), Police National CBRN Centre, CV8 3EN Ryton on Dunsmore, Coventry, UK
e-mail: john.stephenson@wmas.nhs.uk

© Springer International Publishing Switzerland 2015   107
P. Wankhade, K. Mackway-Jones (eds.), *Ambulance Services,*
DOI 10.1007/978-3-319-18642-9_9

The three main blue-light services have separate identities and cultures that are described below:

- The fire and rescue services are very regimented, with a national rank structure and strong command and control. They work as a team. At a major incident, the fire service will have a very robust structured and practiced command and control structure in place as they manage all incidents in the same way; it is just the scale that varies.
- The police forces are mobilised as smaller units of staff that work very well within their team. They tend to have a command structure that manages these smaller teams from a central command facility that is not always at the scene of the incident. Different specialist teams tend to be under different intermediate control structures (e.g. firearms, traffic and forensics) so the middle tier of management of an incident with the police can be quite complicated for other organisations to understand. Working with the police on a single incident could have several scene management teams, often working in silos without oversight of each other's activities.
- The ambulance services over the past 30 years has moved away from the regimented militaristic command structure still present within the fire and police services that is best described as a command and control system as it has become more integrated within the NHS. Within the NHS, teams of staff work under the supervision and guidance of a team leader as opposed to the command of a senior officer. Ambulance staff have the added complication that they largely work as a solo responder or in teams of two clinicians (a paramedic and a supporting clinician working such as an emergency medical technician or emergency care support worker), they are not used to working as part of teams within a command structure. There is also the different nature of work whereby the clinicians have an ultimate responsibility for the care of patients and that can lead to conflict when, in larger incidents, the scene management structure is trying to bring order to the incident and the ambulance staff are focused more on the care of an individual patient rather than the "greater good" of the whole affected population. The NHS is also working in a system of leadership for patient care or incident management where the leadership follows function and not role, so for example, a trauma team consisting of several medical consultants may be led by a more junior member of staff who takes the overall coordination role and leaves the experts to manage their own areas of expertise.

So when trying to develop interoperability between the three blue-light services in the UK, we have different structures, different cultures as well as different organisational boundaries. For example, within the UK, we have 13 ambulance trusts, 45 police forces and 54 fire and rescue services that do not have contiguous boundaries so that, for example, the average ambulance service has to liaise with 5 police and fire services. London, Scotland and Northern Ireland are the only areas which have a single geographical area with the same boundaries for the three emergency services which in theory should provide easier interoperability.

The Need to Change

Following several major incidents, there has been a recurrent theme in the debriefing and public enquiries that the emergency services need to work together more closely limiting duplication and improving outcomes for the public. There has been a need for better interoperability for years, and when this works well it has usually been because of the people on duty on that day, who may have previous contacts or may be more collaborative in their management styles.

In a report commissioned by the Cabinet Office Civil Contingencies Secretariat by the Emergency Planning College, the common causes of failures identified within 38 public enquiry reports (see Appendix 1 for list) that are relevant to interoperability include:

• Poor working practices and organisational planning
• Inadequate training
• Ineffective communication
• Lack of leadership
• Failure to learn lessons

It was decided that interoperability should not be left to chance and so Theresa May, Home Secretary in 2012, started the Joint Emergency Services Interoperability Programme (JESIP) so that interoperability would become the norm and not be the historical exception. The aim of the programme was to achieve better cooperation and coordination between the three emergency services at the scene of a major incident, however, the side effect would be better for day-to-day working between the three services.

Joint Emergency Services Interoperability Programme

Initially, JESIP concentrated on the three major blue-light services of police, fire and ambulance. To change the mind-set and ways of working of thousands of on-scene commanders was a big task for the small tri-service team created and hosted by the Home Office. A particular requirement was not just to solve this problem in England but an acceptance that cross-border mutual aid should also include Scotland, Wales, Northern Ireland and the Channel Islands. By August 2014, all of the devolved administrations apart from Scotland were fully signed up to the JESIP process. The initial stages of the programme were to develop a joint doctrine that the three services could agree upon and that was in accordance with the Civil Contingencies Act 2004 guidance set out in emergency response and recovery. JESIP have adopted the definition of interoperability to be "the extent to which organisations can work together coherently as a matter of routine".

JESIP has been given the task to train commanders, at the operational and tactical levels, however, strategic commanders receive an input through the Multiagency Gold Interoperability Course (MAGIC), which is aligned to JESIP and is delivered through the College of Policing. Following completion, they should be able to demonstrate that they have received appropriate interoperability training in their both preparation and response arrangements to ensure the highest possible levels of joint working. Initially, the training was limited to the three blue-light services, but this also extends to cover those agencies that also respond to emergency situations such as HM Coastguards, other police forces (such as military police, British Transport Police) and also to involve some of the voluntary rescue agencies such as the Royal National Lifeboat Institute (RNLI) and search and rescue organisations such as mountain and cave rescue groups.

Principles for Joint Working

Responders from all agencies involved in decision-making at the incident must apply the principles. This process is to be used when they are determining an appropriate course of action to respond to the threats and hazards associated with the incident and come to a shared understanding of how their different agencies' policies, procedures and relevant legislation are applied to produce a coherent response. They should be reflected in standard operating procedures for joint working in the response to and coordination of an emergency. Some of these principles have developed from other areas of successful joint working on a smaller scale such as the emergency service response to a terrorist firearms incident within the UK.

The principals that have been agreed upon by the JESIP team based within the Home Office are now the backbone of the JESIP doctrine:

1. Co-location
2. Communication
3. Coordination
4. Joint understanding of risk
5. Shared situational awareness

The public expects that the emergency services will work together, particularly in the initial response, to preserve life and reduce harm at any emergency. The purpose of clear, simple principles is to help commanders to take action under pressure that will enable the achievement of successful outcomes. This simplicity is of paramount importance in the early stages of an incident or emergency, when clear, robust decisions and actions need to be taken with minimum delay in an often rapidly changing environment. At the scene, the expected sequence of actions would comprise the first meeting of police, fire and ambulance commanders (co-location); a joint assessment of the situation and prevailing risks (communication, joint risk assessment and shared situational awareness); and a coordinated plan for action.

Below are the agreed definitions and expectations for each of the JESIP principles:

Co-location

Co-location of commanders is essential and allows those commanders to perform the functions of command, control and coordination and face to face, at a single and easily identified location. This is known as the forward command post (FCP), which is a location near to the scene, where the response by the emergency services is managed.

Communication

Communication is the passage of clear, unambiguous and timely information relevant to an emergency situation. Meaningful and effective communication underpins effective joint working. The sharing of information, free of acronyms, across service boundaries is essential to operational success. This starts through pre-planning and between control rooms prior to deployment of resources.

Communication is the capability to exchange reliable and accurate information, that is, critical information about hazards, risks and threats, as well as understanding each organisation's responsibilities and capabilities. The understanding of any information shared ensures the achievement of shared situational awareness that underpins the best possible outcomes of an incident.

The JESIP programme aims to enable emergency responders to use common symbols and terminology and there is an aim that over time there should be convergence of the systems currently in use.

Following judicial review of previous major incidents, a recurrent theme has been the lack of interoperability and communication systems between the three blue-light emergency services and they now share a common communications platform called Airwave that is based on the terrestrial trunked radio (TETRA) digital radio network. It is now possible for all commanders to communicate using a single, secure digital device, sharing talk groups at incidents and still being accessible to their own organisations.

Coordination

Coordination involves the integration of the priorities, resources, decision-making and response activities of each emergency service to avoid potential conflicts, prevent duplication of effort, minimise risk and promote successful outcomes. Effective coordination generally requires one service to act in a "lead" capacity, such as chairing coordination meetings and ensuring an effective response. The lead service will usually be the police service, partly because they can manage access and egress to the incident, but also because often their role at the start of the incident is separate to the roles of patient treatment and hazard management (such as fire) and the police role intensifies once the incident scene is handed over as a crime scene, once all patients are removed and the hazards have been managed. However, in certain circumstances, other services/agencies may be a more appropriate choice, depending upon the nature of the emergency, the phase of the response and the capabilities required.

Joint Understanding of Risk

Risk arises from threats and/or hazards which will be seen, understood and treated differently by different emergency services. This difference in assessing and managing risks is related to the policies, procedures and risk appetite of the organization that is applied in their standard daily activities, which are often very different than when the staff are placed in the centre of a major incident involving multiple casualties and potential ongoing hazards such as the risk of further explosion or secondary devices hidden at an incident designed to harm responders.

In the context of a joint response, sharing information and understanding about the likelihood and potential impact of risks and the availability and implications of potential control measures will ensure, as far as is reasonably practicable, that the agreed aim and objectives are not compromised. This will include ensuring the safety of responders and mitigating the impact of risks on members of the public, infrastructure and the environment. The JESIP doctrine has developed a shared risk management system which follows later in this chapter called the joint decision model (JDM).

Shared Situational Awareness

This is a common understanding of the circumstances and immediate consequences of the emergency, together with an appreciation of the available capabilities and emergency services' priorities. Achieving shared situational awareness is essential for effective interoperability in the emergency response and can be achieved by using METHANE as the standard incident description method and the JDM to come to shared decisions. Both of these are explored more fully later in this chapter. Shared situational awareness relates not only to a common understanding between incident commanders, but also between control rooms and all tiers of the command structure.

The Joint Decision Model

A wide range of decision-making models exist, including specific models used by the individual emergency services. Such models have been developed over several years and have existed to support decision-makers working under difficult circumstances and a guiding principle is that they should not be over complicated. One of the difficulties commanders facing from different organisations in a joint emergency response is how to bring together the available information, reconcile objectives and then make effective decisions together. Prior to the JESIP programme, the fire and rescue service and the police had well-practiced and developed models to support decision-making, but they were different and caused issues around shared decision-making. This led to the development of the JDM, (See Fig. 9.1 for model) taking the best from the decision models currently in use.

In common with most decision-making models, the JDM is organised around three primary considerations, the descriptions are taken from the JESIP doctrine:

Situation: What is happening, what are the impacts, what are the risks, what might happen and what is being done about it? Situational awareness is having an appropriate knowledge of these factors.

Direction: What end state is desired, what are the aims and objectives of the emergency response and what overarching values and priorities will inform and guide this?

Action: what needs to be decided and what needs to be done to resolve the situation and achieve the desired end state?

The JDM develops these considerations and sets out the various stages of how joint decisions should be reached. One of the guiding principles of the JDM is that decision-makers will use their judgement and experience in deciding what additional questions to ask and considerations to take into account, to reach a jointly agreed decision. They must therefore be free to interpret the JDM for themselves, reasonably and according to the circumstances facing them at any given time. Strict adherence to the stepped process outlined in the JDM should always be secondary to achieving desired outcomes, particularly in time-sensitive situations. A detailed and well-practiced understanding of the JDM will facilitate clear and ordered thinking under stress. The following sections summarise the questions and considerations that commanders should think about in following the model.

The JDM can be used for any type of incident from a rapid onset to a rising tide emergency to enable the establishment of shared situational awareness. The advantage of this is that the decision makers are then used to applying a single decision-making model in their day-to-day operational duties and will therefore find it easy to apply in stressful situation of a major incident.

After many years of major incident review identifying the lack of interoperability and cooperation, the UK, emergency services have been undergoing a major change with the intention of interoperability being the expected norm. The JESIP identified that over 10,000 operational and tactical commanders would require training in the new way of working and this is being achieved by each commander attending a day's training, which is delivered by a multiagency team from each of the blue-light services. This has not only significantly increased the understanding of the issues and pressures being experienced by the different services but also forged some of the relationships that over time had started to diminish due to the different organisational pressures that had removed the capacity for commanders to participate in exercises.

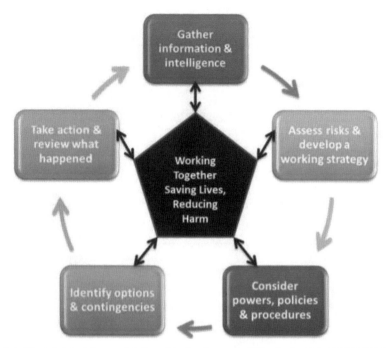

Fig. 9.1 The joint decision model for achieving interoperability in the UK. (JESIP 2014, Joint Doctrine)

An early success was the adoption of METHANE as the single message to be used by each service for declaration of a major incident and communicating the relevant information to the service-specific control room that would then be understood when shared with other services. This has been a big change for the fire and police services but less so for the ambulance services who have been using METHANE for several years.

The METHANE acronym is a standard message:

- M major incident declared (or standby)
- E exact location of incident
- T type of incident
- H hazards (present or potential)
- A access and egress to the scene
- N number of casualties (broken down to severity if possible)
- E emergency services required, and those already in attendance

The success of the training is being verified by a series of exercises where particularly the way the command team interacts is being observed. The challenge will be maintaining the interoperability and not allowing the emergency service to slip back into their silos as staff changes occur over time in those command posts. The success of the JESIP programme will ultimately be measured by how well it becomes a standard practice within the emergency services and no longer needs to be a special strand within command training. The JESIP message has been disseminated through all tiers of the blue-light services with a well organised media strategy and professionally developed supporting training products including an e-learning package that enables the whole response team (from paramedics to chief executives, from volunteer special constables to chief constables and from firefighter to chief fire officers) to be exposed to JESIP ways of working.

Interoperability Outside the UK

The issue of interoperability is very dependent on the organisational structure within each country. In the UK, the police, fire and ambulance services are very separate and the armed forces are rarely called upon to support homeland activities except when a specific issue requiring their skills or manpower is identified.

Looking beyond the UK, it is common for ambulance services to be co-located within the fire services. This is largely a small cadre of staff that responds to the significant traumatic incidents and very sick collapsed patients, and the broader ambulance work is often provided by private organisations rather than as an emergency service. What this means is that there is a much smaller pool of ambulance staff (paramedics) available for a major incident, but they will often already be working as part of the fire service response to that major incident. This then largely leaves two organisations at the major incident in terms of police and fire and these can also sometimes be part of other organisations. For example, in France and Italy, part of the police services (Gendarmerie and Carabinieri) is part of the armed forces. To make the issue more complicated in Italy, there are also local civilian police services so the interoperability may be between the different police units rather than the other emergency services. Therefore, we can assume that interoperability could be an issue with each country depending how they organise their emergency services, how they manage the incident and whether they have preplanned and exercised ways to manage an incident.

Role and Contribution of the National Ambulance Resilience Unit

Prior to the establishment of the JESIP programme, there was sporadic good practice of interoperability. An area that helped demonstrate that interoperability could develop as a result of training, exercising and joint working that was not dependant on individuals was the development of Hazardous Area Response Teams (HART) within the ambulance service. Starting in 2006, HART has rolled out to provide 15 teams across England and Wales with similar teams in Scotland (called Special Operational Response Teams; SORT) and similar capability in Northern Ireland but delivered in a different way where the specialist skills are spread over the response car paramedics rather than concentrated in a specialist unit. The specialist skills include specialist skills and equipment to respond to a Chemical, Biological, Radiological or Nuclear (CBRN) incident, search and rescue skills for a collapsed building, and water rescue skills most likely to be used in flooding incidents. These skills were identified as those required for ambulance staff to work in areas where they had previously not been able to take clinical care due to the extra protective equipment or training required, and it was only by working closely with police and fire colleagues that a training programme developed which allowed patients to be able to benefit from appropriate clinical care and interventions in a more timely manner than previously when they would have needed to be extricated from the incident by fire or police colleagues.

The initial training is coordinated and delivered through the National Ambulance Resilience Unit (NARU) and ongoing skill maintenance and knowledge sharing continues to be an important role in maintaining the UK-wide response to major incidents. A particular example of how NARU were able to develop an interoperable response to a new type of threat was seen following the attack in Mumbai involving several gunmen. It was seen that multiple casualties could be injured in a short time period and that the ambulance response at that stage would struggle to cope with the number of patients. After close working with representatives from the Association of Chief Police Officers (ACPO) and Chief Fire Officers Association (CFOA), a joint approach to risk assessment and clinical treatment proven by joint exercising and training was developed and was seen as the model for what success should look like for the JESIP programme.

Conclusions

The UK has recently tried to bring about significant cultural change within its emergency services with initially promising results. Time will tell if this is maintained, but the benefits in terms of incident management and survivor outcomes are potentially huge. Even at its most basic, the joint organisational learning will be a measure of the legacy of JESIP.

Appendix 1

Year of event	Event
1986	Crowd Safety at Football Grounds
1987	King's Cross Underground Fire
1987	Herald of Free Enterprise
1987	Hungerford Shooting
1988	Piper Alpha Explosion

Year of event	Event
1988	Clapham Rail Crash
1988	Locke rbie Bombing
1989	Hillsborough Stadium Disaster
1989	Kegworth Air Crash
1989/2000	Marchioness–Bowbelle Sinking
1994	Texaco Refinery Explosion
1996	Dunblane Shooting
1996	BSE Outbreak Inquiry
1997	Southall Rail Crash
1997	Stephen Lawrence Murder Inquiry
1999	Ladbroke Grove Rail Inquiry
2000	UK Fuel Disputes
2000	Harold Shipman and 'the 3 Inquiries'
2001/2007	Foot & Mouth Disease
2001	Victoria Climbie Murder
2003	Failures in NHS Report
2003	Bichard Inquiry (Soham Murders)
2004	ICL Factory Explosion
2004	Boscastle Floods
2005	Buncefield Oil Depot Explosion
2005	London Terrorist Attacks
2005	Stockwell Shooting
2005	Carlisle Floods
2007	Hüll Floods
2007	Pitt Review (UK Floods)
2009	Influenza Pandemie
2010	Derrick Bird Shootings

Bibliography

JESIP. (2014). Joint Doctrine: The interoperability framework. www.jesip.org.uk. Accessed Aug. 2014.

National Ambulance Resilience Unit (NARU). (2015). www.naru.org.uk. Accessed Aug. 2014.

Review of Persistent Lessons Identified Relating to Interoperability from Emergencies and Major Incidents since 1986; Dr Kevin Pollock; Emergency Planning College Occasional Papers New Series No. 6, October 2013.

Dr. John Stephenson qualified from the University of Leeds in 1986 and after training posts in Yorkshire became a GP in Belper in Derbyshire in 1993. After working in Medical Management in Primary Care, he became the medical director of East Midlands Ambulance Service in 2006, chaired the UK National Ambulance Medical Directors Group until 2010 and then became the medical director of the National Ambulance Resilience Unit, a role which combines helping plan and train staff for the UK response to major incidents along with strategic advice to the Department of Health and NHS England on emergency preparedness.

Chapter 10
Responding to Diversity and Delivering Equality in Prehospital Care: Statutory Responsibilities, Best Practice and Recommendations

Viet-Hai Phung, Karen Windle and A. Niroshan Siriwardena

Introduction

The population of the UK is becoming increasingly diverse. In England and Wales, the share of the population identifying themselves as from a minority ethnic group rose from 8.7 % to 14.0 % between 2001 and 2011. Within this, the proportion of individuals identifying as Asian or British Asian increased from 4.8 % to 7.5 %, whilst other minority ethnic groups also grew. Indian and Pakistani populations rose from 3.4 to 4.5 % and the population accounted for by Black/African/Caribbean or black British, increased from 2 % to 3.4 %. Following the Accession countries joining the European Union in 2008, there were also significant increases in the White Other population (4 %; Office for National Statistics, ONS 2012). Moving away from a 'heteronormative' view of society, an estimated 2 % to 10 % of the population identify as lesbian, gay or bisexual ((LGB) (Aspinall 2009), although the Integrated Household Survey gave a lower estimate, placing the figure at 1.5 % (ONS 2013a). In the same decade, the number of people aged 65 and over increased by 16 % from 8.3 million to 9.2 million (ONS 2013b). In the next 20 years, the number of those

V.-H. Phung (✉) · K. Windle · A. N. Siriwardena
Community and Health Research Unit, School of Health and Social Care, University of Lincoln, Brayford Campus, Lincoln LN6 7TS, Lincolnshire, UK
e-mail: vphung@lincoln.ac.uk

A. N. Siriwardena
email: nsiriwardena@lincoln.ac.uk

© Springer International Publishing Switzerland 2015
P. Wankhade, K. Mackway-Jones (eds.), *Ambulance Services,*
DOI 10.1007/978-3-319-18642-9_10

aged over 80 years will treble and those over 90 years will double (Greaves and Farbus 2006). These changes in the population profile will increase demands on health,
social and third sector care. For example, the probability of having a long-term condition (LTC) rises with age; some 60 % of those aged 65 years and above reporting
at least one LTC. Those with LTCs account for 50 % of all general practitioner (GP)
appointments, 64 % of outpatient appointments and 70 % of all inpatient bed days
(Department of Health, DH 2012).

Such societal changes are also reflected in the increasing diversity of the National Health Service (NHS) workforce. In 2012, there were around 193,000 staff
from minority ethnic groups in the NHS, constituting 14 % of the total 1.3 million
NHS staff (Kline 2013). A changing age profile is also seen in NHS staff with, for
example, around one in three hospital nurses over the age of 50 years due to retire
soon (Buchan and Seccombe 2012) and future projected shortages of GPs owing to
the ageing workforce (Goodwin 2011).

Population and workforce diversity means that equality is becoming a salient issue for patients or service users and employees. The Equality Act 2010, and within
it, the Public Sector Equality Duty (PSED), is a key legislative response to this
increasing diversity. Within the NHS, the Equality Delivery System (EDS) and its
evolution into EDS2 provides the policy context for equality and diversity issues
(NHS 2012, 2013). As NHS (and public sector) organisations, ambulance services
are bound by the Equality Act 2010, as well as influenced by the EDS and EDS2.
This chapter explores why equality and diversity matter, summarises the Equality
Act (2010) and the PSED, discusses what this means for NHS service users and
staff, and examines what strategic and practice approaches are being undertaken in
the NHS generally, as well as specifically within the ambulance service. The chapter concludes with recommendations for policy and practice.

Why Does Identifying Diversity and Ensuring Equality Matter?

Equality matters because of the unequal service access, treatment and outcomes
reported by minority groups (Hewitson et al. 2014; Moriarty and Manthorpe 2012;
Thomas and Atkinson 2011; Stonewall 2010).

Access to Services

A number of minority groups report unequal access to the services that they need;
either through a lack of knowledge of available services, how these can be appropriately accessed, or their ability to pay. Older people from minority ethnic groups
suffer multiple discrimination (Uccellari 2008). They are more likely to live in poor
quality accommodation or become homeless, both of which can worsen health outcomes. They often have a high need for health and social care support, which is

sometimes unmet due to difficulties in accessing appropriate and necessary services (Blood and Bamford 2010). Research exploring end-of-life care has found that those individuals from higher socioeconomic groups are more likely to die at home due to better knowledge of service availability or referral pathways necessary to access services, and the ability to pay for additional care (Grande et al. 1998). Among disabled older LGB people, 37 % did not access health services compared to 28 % of disabled older heterosexual people. The corresponding figures for social care services were 19 % and 10 %, respectively (Stonewall 2010). In terms of access to care, there are also often gender imbalances, for example, women are less likely to die at home than men. In contrast, more younger women are able to access home care (Grande et al. 1998).

Treatment

Different and sometimes negative experiences of treatment from service providers have been reported by a number of minority groups. For example, 17 % of older lesbian and bisexual women recounted that they had experienced discrimination related to their sexual orientation when using GP services. This compares to 11 % of older gay and bisexual men (Stonewall 2010). Sometimes, this results in an underuse of services with, for example, the social marginalisation of transgender communities leading to a shift away from mainstream services and towards self-help; individuals placing a strong emphasis upon the shared experience (Hines 2007). Evidence also suggests that older patients are less likely to receive the most clinically effective treatment in cancer care (Age UK 2012).

In exploring care given across ambulance services, a recent national quality improvement evaluation found differences in treatment according to sex and age. The Ambulance Services Cardiovascular Quality Initiative (ASCQI) evaluated the effectiveness of implementing a quality improvement collaborative (QIC) for improving ambulance care for acute myocardial infarction (AMI) and stroke. Paramedics in all English ambulance services were trained to apply care bundles for AMI (aspirin, glyceryl trinitrate (GTN), pain assessment and analgesia) and stroke (face–arm–speech test, blood pressure and blood glucose recording; Siriwardena et al. 2014). Using standard regression techniques, men were found to be more likely to receive the AMI care bundle, whilst younger and older individuals were less likely to receive both AMI and stroke care bundles.

Outcomes

In exploring morbidity and mortality, individuals from minority groups have fared less well when compared to the population as a whole. Individuals from minority ethnic groups are up to six times more likely than Whites to suffer from LTCs including diabetes, stroke, chronic obstructive pulmonary disease (COPD), hypertension, depression and anxiety (National Resource Centre for Ethnic Minority Health 2007).

Gypsies and travellers reported difficulties in accessing care leading to a high incidence of early-onset health problems (Blood and Bamford 2010). People with learning difficulties die far younger than the general population (Glover and Ayub 2010). A recent DH-funded inquiry, reported that the median age of death for people with learning disabilities was 65 years for men, compared with 78 years for the UK population and 63 years for women, compared with 83 years for the UK population. Overall, 22% of people with learning disabilities died before the age of 50 years, compared with 9% of the general population (Heslop et al. 2013). Cancer mortality rates have fallen by 16–17% among those under 75 years. However, they rose by 2% among those aged 85 years and over between 1995–1997 and 2003–2005 (UK 2012). Similarly, older people with cancer are less likely to die at home. This may at least partly be related to their poorer access to home care, as well as to services in general (Grande et al. 1998).

Workforce Discrimination

It is not only service users who experience unequal outcomes. There is also substantial evidence of workplace discrimination. For example, in a study of 30 NHS Trusts, a White shortlisted applicant was almost twice as likely to be appointed as a minority ethnic shortlisted applicant (Kline 2013). The 2012 NHS staff survey found that 8% of the workforce had experienced discrimination at work, with 4% citing racial discrimination (Kline 2013). Reports of discrimination among non-white staff had increased from 23% to 26% in the previous 12 months. (up from 23% in 2011). The same survey reported a reduction in discriminatory practices. For example, 17% of disabled staff reported discrimination in the previous 12 months (down from 19% in 2011), whilst 19% of gay male staff (down from 25% in 2011), 14% of lesbian staff (down from 16% in 2011) and 18% of bisexual staff had suffered discrimination (down from 21% in 2011). We have to exercise caution when interpreting the results of the NHS staff survey as only two have been conducted since the Equality Act 2010 became law. The incidence of discrimination needs to be continuously monitored, as does the quality of staff diversity training.

The Equality Act 2010 and the PSED

The concept of equality has evolved over time. Initially, definitions of equality centred on the idea that everybody should have the same access to services and that treatment should be universal. However, in the light of the Equality Act 2010, achieving equality in practice now demands a more proactive role for public bodies. Public bodies now have to consider how they will be, *"addressing disadvantage, accommodating difference, enhancing dignity and facilitating participation"* (Fredman 2011). The Equality Act 2010 unifies and extends previous separate equality legislation, including gender, race and disability. The Act outlaws direct and indirect discrimination, harassment and victimisation of people with relevant protected characteristics in relevant circumstances (NHS 2012). The nine protected characteristics covered by the Act are:

- Age
- Disability
- Gender reassignment
- Marriage and civil partnership
- Pregnancy and maternity
- Race including colour, nationality and ethnic or national origins
- Religion or belief, including a lack of religion or belief, and where belief includes any religious or philosophical belief
- Sex
- Sexual orientation

Section 149 of the Equality Act is the PSED, which harmonises existing equalities legislation by amalgamating the existing gender, race and disability equality duties (Clayton-Hathway 2013; Kline 2013; Colgan and Wright 2011). The PSED consists of the general Equality Duty, which came into force in April 2011 (Section 149 Equality Act 2010), and the specific duties, which became law in September 2011 in England (Kline 2013). The PSED requires public authorities to have

> ...due regard, in the exercise of their functions, to the need to eliminate discrimination, harassment, victimisation and any other conduct prohibited under the 2010 Act, to the need to advance equality of opportunity between persons who share a relevant protected characteristic and persons who do not share it and to the need to foster good relations between such groups. (NHS 2012)

To comply with the PSED, public bodies need to collect, analyse and act upon reliable data around the protected characteristic groups. This is a challenge for the NHS, whose use of data in relation to protected characteristic groups has traditionally been limited in scope and inconsistent in application (Kline 2013; Mathur et al. 2013; Psoinos et al. 2011). Importantly, the legislation confers an obligation on public sector bodies, central government, local authorities and key health sector organisations to continuously monitor their compliance with these duties. Every public body is now required to publish equality objectives at least every four years from 6 April 2012. Information that demonstrates their compliance with those objectives has been published annually from 31 January 2012 (NHS 2012).

Equality and Diversity in the NHS

As public bodies, NHS organisations are bound by the duties set out in The Equality Act 2010 and must aim to comply with the Act's PSED. For NHS organisations, the Equality Delivery System (EDS) and its successor EDS2 provide guidance for complying with their legislative duties.

The Equality Delivery System (EDS)

The EDS was commissioned and steered by the Equality and Diversity Council (EDC). The EDC provides strategic leadership in supporting the NHS to deliver better outcomes for patients, comply with the Equality Act 2010 (in particular, the PSED), as well as ensuring that services and workplaces are personal, equitable and diverse. At all times, the focus of the EDS is on service users and staff. The EDS was formally launched in November 2011 and makes an explicit connection between equality and quality:

> *A quality service is one that recognises the needs and circumstances of each patient, carer, community and staff member, and ensures that services are accessible, appropriate, safe and effective for all, and that workplaces are free from discrimination where staff can thrive and deliver. A service cannot be described as a quality service if only some patients achieve good outcomes while others do not.* (NHS 2012)

The EDS is designed as a toolkit to be applied by the NHS to tackle health inequalities, mitigating socio-economic factors in, "*...the incidence of ill-health, the take-up of treatment and the outcomes from healthcare. In addition, many people from protected groups are challenged by these factors, and as a result, experience difficulties in accessing, using and working in the NHS*" (NHS 2012). However, use of the EDS is voluntary. It provides guidance—rather than statutory targets—that support those organisations across the NHS to achieve their obligations set out in the Equality Act 2010; in particular, those duties set out in the Act's PSED. From the outset, it was envisaged that the EDS would inform the decision-making process, helping with evidence gathering and evaluation of the incidence, prevalence and outcomes associated with protected characteristics. To comply with the PSED, the EDS recommended that organisations should engage with a range of stakeholders: patients, communities and staff (NHS 2012).

The EDS requires each NHS organisation to apply a set of four broad goals encompassing 18 outcomes (see Table 10.1). These goals reflect those issues that are of utmost concern to key stakeholders, including: patients, communities, staff and executive board members. The performance of ambulance services is assessed by these stakeholders against each indicator. The progress that each ambulance service makes is then measured against a four-level colour-coded grading scale, indicating if the organisation is 'underdeveloped', 'developing', 'achieving' or 'excelling' against each outcome. Their progress thein inform decisions about future priority actions needed to be undertaken by the ambulance trust.

Table 10.1 Equality diversity system (EDS) goals

Goal	Description
Better health outcomes for all	The NHS should achieve improvements in patient health, public health and patient safety for all, based on comprehensive evidence of needs and results
Improved patient access and experience	The NHS should improve accessibility and information and deliver the right services that are targeted, useful, usable and used in order to improve the patient experience
Empowered, engaged and well-supported staff	The NHS should increase the diversity and quality of the working lives of the paid and nonpaid workforce, supporting all staff to better respond to patients' and communities' needs
Inclusive leadership at all levels	NHS organisations should ensure that equality is everyone's business, and everyone is expected to take an active part, supported by the work of specialist equality leaders and champions

NHS National Health Service

Implementing and Embedding the EDS

There are a number of steps that each organisation is required to undertake in order to implement and embed the EDS in their organisational structure and delivery:

Step 1: The confirmation of governance arrangements and partnership working
Step 2: Engagement with local interests including patients, communities, staff, staff-side organisations and local voluntary organisations
Step 3: The use of best available evidence
Step 4: Partnership working with local authorities

Implementation starts with step 1, whilst steps 2–4 can occur simultaneously. The process of embedding the EDS starts with collaborating with local stakeholders to analyse performance against the four goals and 18 outcomes (see Table 10.1). The evidence gathered at step 3 is shared with all stakeholders and the performance of the trust is analysed. Having shared the evidence, an overall grade is agreed for each outcome, accounting for variations between protected groups and performance across sites and services. The results of these analyses form a significant part of the information that organisations are required to publish annually in compliance with the PSED. Starting with the grades agreed across all 18 outcomes (i.e., 'underdeveloped', 'developing', 'achieving' or 'excelling'), local stakeholders and the organisation then select four or five equality objectives to be addressed for the coming business planning period. Ambulance services need to prioritise since there is evidence that not all protected groups have the same need for treatment, nor are services delivering outcomes with the same level of effectiveness. The collation, analysis and discussion of evidence around protected groups should define the highest priorities, enabling an action or activity plan to be developed. Failure to prioritise could lead to half-hearted attempts to address all the protected groups' needs instead of taking concerted action with those that are facing the highest levels of discrimination, or poorest outcomes (NHS 2012). Prioritisation does not mean that some protected groups will be sidelined. It is likely that prioritising core objectives will include a range of minority groups during the four-year lifetime of the delivery plan (NHS 2012).

The priority objectives are then integrated into the organisation's business plan. All organisations are statutorily required to publish their 'grades' and equality objectives in their annual reports. It is recommended that ongoing progress is shared with Health and Wellbeing Boards (based in local authorities) with a view to possible future joint action. Providers may highlight and discuss their equality objectives and rate of progress with commissioners as part of any agreed contract monitoring processes (NHS 2012).

The Evolution to EDS2

In November 2013, EDS2 was launched. On top of the original remit of the EDS, this new framework encourages flexibility to reflect particular local needs and concerns. It also supports sharing good practice between organisations where possible (NHS 2013). EDS2 develops the socio-economic underpinning of health inequalities (NHS 2012; Malmivaara 2014; NHS 2013), recognised by the original EDS (NHS 2012), by expanding the list of protected groups where concerted action is needed to improve access and outcomes (NHS 2013). Along with the nine protected characteristic groups covered by the Equality Act 2010, EDS2 now applies to the following groups:

- People who are homeless
- People who live in poverty
- People who are long-term unemployed
- People in stigmatised occupations (such as women and men involved in prostitution)
- People who misuse drugs
- People with limited family or social networks
- People who are geographically isolated (NHS 2013)

Good Practice in the NHS

Progress towards equality has been varied (Clayton-Hathway 2013), although good practice exemplars are available. For example, NHS trusts across Airedale, Bradford and Leeds worked with their voluntary and community sectors to improve evidence collection and use this to inform objectives and service delivery (Clayton-Hathway 2013). To improve services directed towards LGB or transgender communities, Oxleas NHS Foundation Trust introduced monitoring data on the sexual orientation of service users to support the identification of health needs and delivery of targeted and appropriate service provision. Initial data collection identified a lack of confidence among staff about asking users to disclose their sexual orientation. An e-learning package was then created to enable and support staff in requesting such sensitive information from patients and raise awareness about LGB health inequalities (Clayton-Hathway 2013). Nevertheless, the varied nature of progress towards embedding those actions required by the Equality Act 2010 means that there will be cases where public bodies have not achieved the same standards.

Progress Towards Identifying Diversity and Achieving Equality in the Ambulance Service

Case Studies

As we have already discussed, the EDS and EDS2 are voluntary and each ambulance service needs to decide how they will deliver the PSED and requirements under the Equality Act 2010. As such, there will inevitably be variations in the strategies adopted and the extent to which ambulance services progress towards compliance. For example, in relation to the requirement that the equality objectives are published, some ambulance services have chosen to publish information on all four goals (see Table 10.1) once every four years, whilst others have chosen to publish annually. This variability makes it difficult to compare progress across all ambulance services. Similarly, as only some ambulance services have chosen to adopt EDS2 (which had only been operational, at the time of writing, for a matter of months), no published data are available. To better understand the process and progress, two case studies are provided below. The first explores the actions of South Central Ambulance Service (SCAS) in adopting the EDS, whilst the second discusses the early progress of East Midlands Ambulance Service (EMAS) in applying EDS2 (Personal communication, Barot, M., 20 February 2014).

Case Study: South Central Ambulance Service NHS Trust (SCAS) and the Equality Delivery System (EDS)
South Central Ambulance Service NHS Trust (SCAS) chose to adopt the EDS. All four goals were assessed in four separate stakeholder events spread over the whole of the SCAS catchment area. Each included representatives from the nine protected characteristic groups. The representatives were selected by Milton Keynes Equalities Council, Community Action Hampshire and Slough Council for Voluntary Service, all of whom had service-level agreements with SCAS. The workforce assessments, goals three and four 'empowered, engaged and well-supported staff' and 'inclusive leadership at all levels' were made by union representatives and staff.
SCAS was judged to have done very well against the first goal 'better health outcomes for all' where not only five outcomes but also 31 foci were assessed. Of these 31 foci, they were assessed to be 'achieving' in 21 and

'excelling' in eight (SCAS 2012). Four outcomes and 24 foci were assessed in the second goal of Improving patient access and experience. SCAS was assessed to be 'achieving' in 18 foci and 'developing' in the other six (SCAS 2012).

There were six outcomes with a total of 35 foci to be considered and graded in the third goal 'empowered, engaged and included staff'. On 23 of the 35 foci, SCAS was assessed to be 'achieving', whilst in five, they were 'excelling' (SCAS 2012). On the fourth goal of 'inclusive leadership at all levels', there were three outcomes and 14 foci. Of these foci, SCAS were 'achieving' in nine and 'developing' in the other five (SCAS 2012). All goals, outcomes and foci are subject to an annual review.

SCAS has taken tangible action to improve outcomes for members of protected characteristic communities. For patients whose first language is not English, SCAS provides a language line service and have now introduced a 41 language phrasebook to all staff and patients. They have also worked with British Telecom to ensure that patients with communication difficulties, speech or hearing impairments can access type and talk. SCAS provides training for staff to appropriately work alongside patients with learning disability and are currently engaging with Gypsy and Traveller communities to identify and train community first responders from fixed sites across the counties (SCAS 2012).

Despite the impressive assessment ratings provided by stakeholders and staff, SCAS recognises that more progress is necessary if they are to achieve equality for service users and staff. In particular, there is a need to improve data collection; some monitoring data were patchy with more data being available for some protected characteristic groups than others. Engagement with representatives from the protected characteristic groups was also considered to be uneven when set against some goals, outcomes and foci (SCAS 2012).

Case Study: East Midlands Ambulance Service NHS Trust (EMAS) and Equality Delivery System 2 (EDS2)

East Midlands Ambulance Service NHS Trust (EMAS) has chosen to adopt the EDS2 pathway towards equality and diversity. As EDS2 was only implemented in November 2013, it is too early at this stage, to draw definitive conclusions about EMAS' progress or otherwise towards their objectives. So, inevitably, they do not yet have published results in relation to their progress against the four main goals and 18 outcomes (see Table 10.1).

However, EMAS has undertaken a number of actions. They have extensively engaged with local stakeholders, including the general public, voluntary and community groups. EMAS has also organised a meeting of Chairs from all of the former Local Involvement Networks (LINs). Sessions have profiled the EDS2 and attempted to gain a baseline assessment score. However, representatives felt they needed more time and information to 'grade' the Trust. Service users felt they had received little information and their lack of any prior or ongoing engagement resulted in the delay in any 'grading' exercise.

Despite EMAS' efforts to engage with local stakeholders, levels of attendance by representatives from protected characteristic communities were disappointing. Such poor attendance was attributed to an incomplete database of contacts and choice of venues. Resource issues have been cited as a barrier to more effective engagement with local stakeholders.

Currently, the Trust collates workforce data across the protected characteristics. This includes recording the number of grievance or disciplinary procedures, flexible working, complaints around bullying and harassment. Some data are collected to support staff education and training, but this does not extend across all protected characteristic groups. Data collection is also incomplete in relation to the number of patients who have protected characteristics. This paucity of data has affected the extent to which EMAS can appropriately engage their stakeholders; the organisation is unaware of how to access, invite and involve different communities. EMAS staff have yet to embed the processes of EDS2 in practice; many of the requirements are seen as peripheral to their ongoing pressures of work. Further strategies, structures and processes (including appropriate data collection, outreach work and engagement) need to be implemented if EDS2 is to be effectively and universally implemented.

Continuing Issues with the EDS and EDS2

Data collection and monitoring are essential if the EDS and EDS2 are to be appropriately delivered. However, despite these toolkits and the Equality Act 2010 raising the profile of protected communities as service users and providers, awareness of their problems in relation to access to, treatment and outcomes from, services is still patchy (Moriarty and Manthorpe 2012). There is inconsistent quality and usage of data on the different protected characteristic groups between ambulance services. Some ambulance services lack sufficient quantity and quality of data across all communities, whilst others lack data on particular protected characteristic groups. Monitoring for race and ethnicity is now at acceptable levels following introduction of the public sector race equality legislation. However, monitoring of disability generally contains large gaps, and the monitoring of sexual orientation is non-existent (Ali et al. 2013).

As the two case studies above illustrate, engagement with stakeholders has varied between ambulance services. EDS2 gives flexibility for each to prioritise particular local concerns, which will then be reflected in the types of stakeholders with which they engage (NHS 2013). Whilst this has the advantage of reflecting local priorities and needs, it makes the task of comparing best practice across ambulance services very difficult.

Recommendations

In response to the ongoing issues with EDS and EDS2, it is recommended that ambulance services should share best practice, where possible, in the following areas:

- *Data collection and usage.* Ambulance services with a strong evidence base in particular protected characteristic groups need to share their good practice (e.g. how they approached particular communities, staff training in asking sensitive questions, publicity, etc.) with those organisations that are struggling to identify and gather data from the same communities.
- *Engaging local stakeholders.* The requirements and scoring of EDS and EDS2 must be publicised far more widely through existing community groups, outreach work needs to be carried out and individuals proactively recruited to ensure representative and appropriate engagement. Venues to which individuals are invited need to be accessible. Consideration should also be given to organising transport to enable attendance, whilst payment for travel and users time should also be provided.
- *Staff and union engagement.* Staff need to be actively encouraged to perceive the EDS as a mechanism to improve their practice—rather than as (yet another) bureaucratic, top-down, 'tick-box' demand. To deliver the effective and appropriate treatment necessary to improve health outcomes, the different needs and sensitivities of particular communities need to be understood and met.

Conclusion

The Equality Act 2010 and PSED have had a significant impact on the way that public sector organisations are required to operate in relation to their staff and service users. Public sector organisations now have a duty to proactively pursue equality in response to the increasing diversity of the population they serve and the staff that work for them. The EDS and its successor EDS2 are voluntary approaches within the NHS designed to ensure that their organisations comply with the legislative duties, set out in the PSED of the Equality Act 2010. Partly because of the early stages of implementing the EDS, and especially EDS2, there is a dearth of published information about the extent to which organisations in the NHS and in particular, ambulance services are progressing towards their equality objectives. Data collection and analysis has been variable across the protected characteristic groups and ambulance services, which makes the sharing best practice difficult. Ambulance services adopting different approaches and service responses also hinders the extent to which best practice can be shared. Whilst local flexibility is a positive feature of the EDS and EDS2 in particular, some standardisation of approaches maybe needed to drive forward the equalities agenda.

Acknowledgments Our thanks to Ludlow Johnson and Mukesh Barot, equality and diversity managers for SCAS and EMAS, respectively, who provided invaluable information that formed the basis for the two case studies in this chapter.

References

Age UK, Department of Health, & MacMillan Cancer Support. (2012). *Cancer services coming of age: Learning from the improving cancer treatment assessment and support for older people project*. London: Department of Health.

Ali, S., Burns, C., & Grant, L. (2013). Equality and diversity in the health service. *Journal of Psychological Issues in Organizational Culture, 3*(S1), 190–209.

Aspinall, P. J. (2009). *Estimating the size and composition of the lesbian, gay and bisexual population in Britain. Research report 37*. Manchester: Equality and Human Rights Commission.

Blood, I., & Bamford, S. (2010). *Equality and diversity and older people with high support needs*. York: Joseph Rowntree Foundation.

Buchan, J., & Seccombe, I. (2012). Using scenarios to assess the future supply of NHS nursing staff in England. *Human resources for Health, 10*(16), 1–9.

Clayton-Hathway, K. (2013). *The public sector equality duty—Analysis of supporting evidence*. Oxford: Centre for Diversity Policy Research and Practice.

Colgan, F., & Wright, T. (2011). Lesbian, gay and bisexual equality in a modernizing public sector 1997–2010: Opportunities and threats. *Gender, Work & Organization, 18*(5), 548–570.

Department of Health (DH). (2012). *Long term conditions compendium of information* (3rd ed.). London: Department of Health.

Fredman, S. (2011). The public sector equality duty. *Industrial Law Journal, 40*(4), 405–427.

Glover, G., & Ayub, M. (2010). *How people with learning disabilities die*. Lancaster: Learning Disabilities Observatory.

Goodwin, N. (2011). *Improving the quality of care in general practice: Report of an independent inquiry commissioned by the King's Fund*. London: King's Fund.

Grande, G., Addington-Hall, J., & Todd, C. (1998). Place of death and access to home care services: Are certain patient groups at a disadvantage? *Social Science Medicine, 47*(5), 565–579.

Greaves, C. J., & Farbus, L. (2006). Effects of creative and social activity on the health and wellbeing of socially isolated older people: Outcomes from a multi-method observational study. *The Journal of the Royal Society for the Promotion of Health, 126*(3), 134–142.

Heslop, P., Blair, P., Fleming, P., Hoghton, M., Marriott, A., & Russ, L. (2013). *Confidential inquiry into premature deaths of people with learning disabilities (CIPOLD)*. Bristol: Norah Fry Research Centre.

Hewitson, P., Skew, A., Graham C., Jenkinson, C., & Coulter, A. (2014). People with limiting long-term conditions report poorer experiences and more problems with hospital care. *BMC Health Services Research, 14*(33), 1–10.

Hines, S. (2007). Transgendering care: Practices of care within transgender communities. *Critical Social Policy, 27*(4), 462–486.

Kline, R. (2013). *Discrimination by appointment: How black and minority ethnic applicants are disadvantaged in NHS staff recruitment*. London: Public World.

Malmivaara, A. (2014). On decreasing inequality in health care in a cost-effective way. *BMC Health Services Research, 14*(79), 1–4.

Mathur, R., Grundy, E., & Smeeth, L. (2013). *Availability and use of UK based ethnicity data for health research. Working paper 01/13.* London: National Centre for Research Methods.

Moriarty, J., & Manthorpe, J. (2012). *Diversity in older people and access to services—An evidence review.* London: Age UK.

National Resource Centre for Ethnic Minority Health. (2007). *A guide to working with black and minority ethnic communities in Scotland living with long term conditions.* Glasgow: National Resource Centre for Ethnic Minority Health.

NHS. (2012). *The equality delivery system for the NHS—Making sure everyone counts.* London: NHS.

NHS. (2013). *A refreshed Equality Delivery System for the NHS: EDS2—Making sure everyone counts.* London: NHS.

Office for National Statistics (ONS). (2012). *Ethnicity and national identity in England and Wales 2011.* London: ONS.

Office for National Statistics (ONS). (2013a). *Key findings from the Integrated Household Survey: January 2012 to December 2012 (Experimental Statistics).* London: ONS.

Office for National Statistics (ONS). (2013b). *What does the 2011 Census tell us about older people?* London: ONS.

Psoinos, M., Hatzidimitriadou, E., Butler, C., & Barn, R. (2011). *Ethnic monitoring in healthcare services in the UK as a mechanism to address health disparities: A narrative review.* London: Swan IPI.

South Central Ambulance Service (SCAS). (2012). *Equality delivery system 2012–2016.* Bicester: South Central Ambulance Service.

Siriwardena, A. N., Shaw, D., Essam, N., Togher, F. J., Davy, Z., Spaight, A., et al. (2014). The effect of a national quality improvement collaborative on prehospital care for acute myocardial infarction and stroke in England. *Implementation Science, 9*(17), 1–9.

Stonewall. (2010). *Lesbian, gay and bisexual people in later life.* London: Stonewall.

Thomas, B., & Atkinson, D. (2011). Improving health outcomes for people with learning disabilities. *Nursing Standard, 26*(6), 33–36.

Uccellari, P. (2008). Multiple discrimination: How law can reflect reality. *The Equal Rights Review, 1,* 24–49.

Viet-Hai Phung BA (Hons), MSc (Hons) is a research assistant in the Community and Health Research Unit (CaHRU) at the University of Lincoln. His area of interest is in prehospital care, particularly in the development of outcome measures for ambulance services and prehospital care and outcomes for minority groups.

Dr Karen Windle BA (Hons), MSc, PhD is a reader in health and leads the Older People and Well-Being Programme in Community and Health Research Unit (CaHRU) at the University of Lincoln. Her research activities are to evaluate the effectiveness and cost-effectiveness of interventions or services directed towards older people including prevention, personalisation and measurement of outcomes. Karen has led or been involved in a number of high-profile large scale effectiveness and cost-effectiveness evaluations funded by the UK Department of Health. She has also provided supporting evidence to policymakers, including the Treasury Department, leading to an identification of costs and benefits of preventative services to support older people.

A. Niroshan Siriwardena MBBS, MMedSci, PhD, FRCGP is a professor of Primary and Pre-Hospital Health Care and director of the Community and Health Research Unit (CaHRU) at the University of Lincoln. He trained in medicine at St Bartholomew's Hospital, London, and in research at Nottingham and De Montfort Universities. He is a practising GP whose research focuses on improving healthcare quality and outcomes in general practice, primary care and ambulance services. He leads an NIHR programme, Prehospital Outcomes for Evidence Based Evaluation (PhOEBE). He is funded by grants from the National Institute for Health Research, UK Research Councils and European Commission.

Chapter 11
Dealing with the Austerity Challenge

Robert Till and Anthony Marsh

Introduction

Austerity is a term used in economics to describe government policies which are designed to reduce spending and budgets during adverse economic conditions. Blyth (2013) describes austerity as a form of voluntary deflation in which the economy adjusts through the reduction of wages, prices and public spending to restore competitiveness, which is best achieved by cutting the state's budget, debts and deficits.

Whilst the current government has implemented an austerity policy, it is important to note that the National Health Service (NHS) is receiving more investment than ever before. In the 2008–2009 NHS report, Sir David Nicholson, the then NHS chief executive, sets out the 'Nicholson challenge'. This challenge, through the implementation of the Quality, Innovation, Productivity and Prevention (QUIPP) programme, instructed the NHS to deliver efficiency savings of £ 15–20 billion between 2011 and 2014. The efficiency savings are not direct cuts to budgets, but a method of creating £ 15–20 billion more value from the current budget.

An ambulance service now has to do more with less, particularly those ambulance services that hold NHS Foundation Trust status. A foundation trust has to be run as a business. The board of directors has to guarantee a continuity of service and operate as a going concern, whereby it guarantees to pay its bills and debts as laid out in Monitor's Risk Assessment Framework. Monitor is the regulatory body

R. Till (✉)
West Midlands Ambulance Service NHS FT, Trust HQ, Waterfront Business Park,
Waterfront Way, Brierley Hill DY5 1LX, West Midlands, UK
e-mail: Robert.Till@wmas.nhs.uk

A. Marsh
West Midlands Ambulance Service NHS FT, Executive Office, Trust HQ,
Waterfront Business Park, Waterfront Way, Brierley Hill DY5 1LX,
West Midlands, UK
e-mail: Anthony.Marsh@wmas.nhs.uk

© Springer International Publishing Switzerland 2015
P. Wankhade, K. Mackway-Jones (eds.), *Ambulance Services,*
DOI 10.1007/978-3-319-18642-9_11

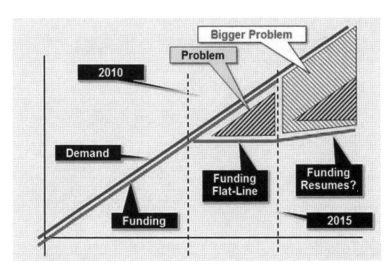

Fig. 11.1 The NHS funding gap (2010–2020). (Lilley 2013)

for foundation trusts. If a trust cannot manage its budget or provide the correct level of service, it will go out of business. To achieve this, the board of directors sets out the target surplus it plans to achieve as part of its 2-year operational plan within the context of a 5-year strategic plan.

Figure 11.1 includes 3a graph illustrating the financial challenge faced by the current NHS context.

As can be seen above, demand rises every year. Until 2010, funding was increased to attempt to meet the rise in demand, but this then flatlined in 2010, and the NHS had to create its own efficiencies to release access to the additional money. It is unclear what will happen in 2015 regarding funding. It is, however, very unlikely that funding will match demand. If demand does continue to rise at its historical rate, then after 2015 the NHS will have to at least double its efficiencies to fill the gap in funding.

The critical question is whether this is possible. As ambulance services have already had to streamline its operations and structure and create efficiencies between 2010 and 2015, how will a trust create the necessary efficiencies between 2015 and 2020. Pre-hospital, community care and commissioning arrangements will have to change radically to enable such efficiency savings.

Changes in Attitude and Demographics

Within the NHS, austerity measures are being further compounded by the change in demographics. The increasing proportion of elderly in our population places ambulance services under increased pressure. The Lords Committee on Public Service and Demographic Change (House of Lords 2012) cited figures from the Office for National Statistics that forecast a 50 % rise in the number of patients over 65's and a doubling in patients over 85's between 2010 and 2030.

A significant proportion of ambulance responses are to assist elderly patients. Some of the most common types of calls include:

- Assisting the frail elderly who have fallen out of bed uninjured, but are unable to assist themselves back up
- Treatment and transport of an elderly patient who has fallen and suffered a traumatic injury requiring hospital treatment and/or admission
- Primary care-related medical conditions or exacerbation of a chronic medical condition

Ambulance services also respond to an increasing number of psychiatric- and social-related problems. Patients who have self-harmed or are having suicidal thoughts often rely upon the ambulance service for assistance. These cases can prove difficult for paramedics to deal with as transport to a hospital emergency department may not be required, and getting assistance from suitably trained professionals can be difficult to arrange, especially out of hours. A similar problem exists with patients who call because of social reasons, although they need help the ambulance service is limited in what support they can provide and can spend excessive lengths of time on scene arranging support meaning that they are not available to respond to other emergencies.

Various measures have been employed to deal with these types of cases by improving relationships with our partners. These include working more closely with the police, general practitioners (GPs) and safeguarding colleagues.

- Ambulance staff are encouraged to make a vulnerable adult safeguarding referrals for those patients who are at risk from further harm or self-neglect.
- Alternate response vehicles which may be used for cases where a patient has fallen over in their home and are unable to get back up, however, are uninjured. These patients do not require a double crewed paramedic ambulance. There may be a multidisciplinary vehicle such as a GP and paramedic or a police officer, paramedic and psychiatric nurse. These resources can be targeted to the calls where patients maybe ordinarily be transported to hospital because no alternative can be found. The GP may provide medication or a prescription that the paramedic cannot and the psychiatric nurse will be able to refer directly to mental health services.

Due to improvements in medical and social care, people can survive longer from chronic conditions or actually be successfully treated and discharged from previously fatal acute episodes, whether that be medical or traumatic in origin.

Attitudes towards healthcare have also seen changes; there is now greater emphasis on the principle of wellbeing and holistic care. Historically, people would only seek medical assistance when it was absolutely necessary. If they were not embarrassed, then they certainly did not want to 'bother the doctor'. The ambulance service was definitely a last resort and was only called if there really was no other option. (Foster et al. 2001) stated:

> Help was only sought when it was considered absolutely necessary. The stoicism was felt to reflect the shared values of 'our generation' and the experience of having to pay to see a doctor prior to the establishment of the NHS.

With increased health awareness, people are now far more likely to visit their GP for investigations. There is also an attitude that there must be a medical solution, no matter what your symptoms. This combined with people working for much longer hours, means that the relatively new out-of-hours services are being utilised more than ever. This has had an impact on the NHS and local government.

The role of the ambulance service has changed too. People no longer just call an ambulance if they have life-threatening complaints that render them unable to get to the hospital themselves. The public will call upon the ambulance service for a multitude of reasons. This could be because they are unsure who else can help them. Hopefully, with the introduction of services such as 111 (a free NHS telephone triage-based signposting service), these occurrences will be reduced. Patients are sometimes identified as needing to attend an emergency department, but do not require an emergency ambulance. However, due to ease, lack of other transport or even because it is a common assumption, people think you can be seen straight away if transported by ambulance—they dial 999.

By improving triage, training clinical staff to make more detailed assessments and jointly working with other healthcare providers to develop alternate pathways of care, both ambulance responses to incidents and the need to convey patients to a hospital could be reduced.

Is Austerity the Catalyst for Innovation?

To create efficiencies, ambulance service leaders, and indeed, the NHS and partner organisations have had to think differently and adapt many of their processes. Some of these could include:

Using Resources to Maximum Efficiency

Traditionally, ambulance services operated by ensuring responding ambulances were mobilised out of an ambulance station, where there could be a varying number of vehicles and varying styles of rota. Usually, the number of ambulances operating out of that station would remain similar on a day-by-day and hour-of-the-day basis. The rotas may have had different start and finish times and are operated for 8-, 10- or 12-h shifts. An ambulance crew would be deployed to an emergency call from the station and then on completion of the incident be returned to their ambulance station where they would wait to receive the next call.

This model was deemed inefficient for several reasons. First, having a set number of ambulances on duty meant that during quieter periods, there was a chance that ambulance crews will remain at the station and on standby, consequently not actually working. Second, having staff and ambulances return to 'their' station meant that some areas may have shortage of ambulances and others may have several ambulances available. For example, three ambulances in town A could be dealing with emergency calls, but, in town B, there were three ambulances available at the station. When the next emergency call is received in town A, the ambulance has to respond from town B which increases the response time and potentially puts the patient at risk.

Creating a performance cell (as discussed earlier in Chap. 8) makes it possible to forecast demand profiles using historical data and also forecast the areas in which emergency calls are most likely to be received hour by hour. This makes it conceivable to plan rotas and match the number of ambulance crews to the expected number of calls. It then allows ambulance control staff to deploy ambulances to standby areas in the order of the forecast priority.

To make the most of this, a new efficient ambulance model has been adopted by several services. This was explained in more detail in the chapter titled 'Modernising Ambulance Services'.

Aligning Hospital and Pre-hospital Specialist Care

Acute hospital trusts have undergone a reconfiguration of services. Not all hospitals provide the same specialist care. This has an impact on ambulance services, as not all patients are now transported to the nearest Emergency Department. Most notably are patients who have suffered from serious trauma, cerebrovascular accident (CVA, stroke) or myocardial infarction (MI, heart attack). Traditionally, patients suffering from these conditions would have been transported to their nearest acute hospital, where they would receive the necessary treatment. If that treatment was unable to be carried out at this hospital, then the patient would be stabilised and then transferred to another hospital for more specialist care.

However, following the reconfiguration of hospitals, specialist acute centres provide the specific care required for each of these patient groups and the local emergency department or hospital trust may not. This reconfiguration reduces the duplication of services within an area and therefore reduces overall costs. As a result, ambulance services have had to adapt the way they operate as the specialist care centre which can treat the patient may not be the nearest hospital. To care for patients during the increased journey times to these centres, paramedics have received extra training and new equipment, and drug regimens have been introduced. This example shows that the NHS as a whole has saved money because services at hospitals are not duplicated; however, because of the extra training and equipment as well as the increased cost associated with longer journeys, the cost to the ambulance service has been increased.

Prioritising and Developing Rigorous Processes

To create the efficiencies required, every department within the ambulance service has had to prioritise and carry out a detailed analysis of its processes. Heads of department are required to do more with less. Services provided, procurement and organisational structure, including staffing levels, are all factors that need streamlining to make sure they are cost effective.

It may be necessary for directors to hold regular meetings with heads of department to refocus and challenge the efficiency drive. The savings made in each department can then be monitored and realigned at a strategic level, which should increase savings and ensure that foundation trusts are succeeding.

Occasionally, an ambulance service may need to spend money in order to save money in the long term. For instance, investing in information technology (IT) infrastructure may be expensive; however, it is probably necessary to improve service and mitigate risk. Likewise, purchasing or renting new property for standby locations, as part of the hub and spoke model, may initially be expensive, but this outlay cost will save money in the long term, as large older ambulance stations are expensive to maintain.

Strategy for Prevention

There is a basis to argue that an increased percentage of money should be spent on health promotion and prevention. If the NHS invested heavily in promoting good health and wellbeing, it may reduce the cost of managing disease to a level which justifies the increased health education expenditure.

For instance, a single visit to a GP on its own is not a large cost to the NHS, but there could be a knock-on effect. If a patient attends a GP out-of-hours appointment for a minor ailment that could have been self-diagnosed and self-treated that GP will not be available to see a patient who may be in greater need. As a result, the second patient may decide to call an ambulance as they have been unsuccessful in gaining an appointment. The ambulance is unable to treat the patient because they require medication not carried by a paramedic, and, because the GP appointments are all full, he or she may have to transport that patient to an emergency department. So in this hypothetical instance, the cost of a single visit to the GP has created the need to pay for an emergency ambulance response and admission into a hospital emergency department.

Examples of different practices exist in other parts of the world and other discipline areas. In Cuba, there is considerably less investment in healthcare than in other countries worldwide, but clinical outcomes are better, despite the per capita spend on healthcare being significantly lower; life expectancy is similar to the USA, but with healthcare costs 96 % lower (Fitz 2011; Campion and Morrissey 2013).

The UK Fire Service has also seen success in concentrating on fire prevention and education, so much so, that it is very rare for a death to occur due to fire. Fire crews spend such little time actually fighting fires as a result of their successful fire prevention campaigns. Fire crews spend a significant proportion of their time based in the community, fitting and checking smoke alarms and offering fire safety advice. If more money was allocated from existing budgets to undertake health promotion and disease screening/prevention, the ambulance service might see a reduction in call demand and consequent costs.

Lack of Control Over Internal and External Factors

There are many external factors and some internal factors that are out of ambulance services control and have a direct effect on ambulance service expenditure. Internally, the Agenda for Change (NHS pay-structure) pay increments that staff are assessed and awarded for each year has a significant cost implication. On average, an employee can expect an increment rise of around £ 800–1500, depending upon their position within a pay band. This means there can be multimillion pound salary increases when the increments are multiplied across an organisation as large as a regional ambulance service. It is vital that an ambulance trust recognises and plans the future workforce. Costs such as continued professional education, education and even the costs associated with longevity in post and an ageing workforce need to be taken into account.

A significant external factor is the cost of fuel, particularly diesel. The ambulance services' primary function and core business is responding quickly to patients. As a result, significant quantities of diesel are purchased. As the number of incidents the ambulance service responds to, and journey distances are increased, due to the transformation of acute hospitals and speciality hospitals, the cost of operating vehicles has increased. This is also compounded when the cost of oil or duty is increased.

These costs can be reduced, but not significantly by bunkering fuel or using fuel cards. Having a means of storing and refuelling vehicles at our own estate means that diesel can be purchased in bulk, and therefore purchased at a reduced cost per litre compared to the commercial forecourt price. Using a fuel card can also mean discounted rates of fuel. A fuel card company will apply a discount to the fuel bill, as they will have negotiated discounted rates with the petrol station companies. This discount is not currently as big as when fuel is bought in bulk by an ambulance service.

As well as vehicle fuel costs, energy to operate control rooms, ambulance stations, response posts and headquarters' buildings also rises with cost implications. Increased costs in energy to run estate can have significant cost implications, especially during long spells of cold weather when heating is used more extensively.

Fig. 11.2 Neoclassical economic theory—supply and
demand curve. (Pilkington
2013)

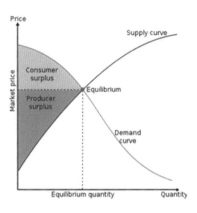

Value of the Ambulance Services

The current commissioning arrangements for ambulance services mean that service providers are paid for the activity they should experience. Each UK taxpayer contributes towards the ambulance service. For example, in 2012, the residents of the West Midlands contributed roughly £ 31.88 per person towards the ambulance service. (This figure is derived by dividing the cost of West Midlands Ambulance Service; WMAS by the population of the West Midlands.) In comparison to other services, for example, considering that a car owner might pay in the region of £ 90 per year for vehicle roadside assistance, the potential life-saving service a resident may receive from the ambulance service makes the £ 31.88 seem proportionally low.

There is a philosophical and perhaps ethical question around the value people place in the ambulance service. Value, as considered here, is demonstrated in the neoclassical economic theory at the equilibrium point below. To put the graph into context, it is worth considering the supply and purchase of plasma TVs. Initially, the new TVs had been very expensive and were not sold in great numbers. This was because the public did not equate the price to the value of the TV. As the price of the TVs came down, they reached a point where they sold in great numbers. This was where the value of the TV matched its price (Fig. 11.2).

If the 'Market Price' axis was replaced with 'Contribution to Ambulance Service' and used the 'Quantity' axis to measure the amount of people, it is interesting to note where the 'Equilibrium' point might be? Perhaps it would be higher than £ 31.88.

Does Commissioning Need to Change?

Currently, local clinical commissioning groups (CCGs), which include the local clinicians, have great powers and responsibility for making commissioning decisions on behalf of their patients and population. It is possible that in times of austerity, there is a need to change the commissioning arrangements to increase value for money. Ethical commissioning is looked at in detail in Chap. 5; however, there are options other than the arrangements in place today which could be considered.

One new approach to commissioning could involve awarding the entire out-of-hospital care for a single patient to one healthcare provider. The job of that provider would be ultimately to keep that patient out of hospital to contain overall costs of medical care.

Currently, a patient may require several healthcare providers to support them. For example, a patient could have healthcare workers going in several times a day for support; he or she may call upon the ambulance service several times a week, and they may also require a district nurse to attend. In the long term, this is expensive; also, because there are so many agencies involved and often they will not be communicating with each other regularly, patients can end up in emergency departments more frequently because the provider is unable to, for whatever reason, solve the current problem in the community and has to resort to calling for an ambulance.

An example of how this approach could work is that Patient A over a period of 12 months costs the NHS £ 300,000 to care for. If a single provider were to be given £ 150,000 to care for that patient, then they would certainly have to think outside the box to achieve the necessary level of care without overspending and reducing possible surplus.

It is, therefore, possible with some restructuring that an ambulance service could become the specialist care provider for out-of-hospital patients. To do this, an ambulance service would need to co-ordinate other community providers to deliver the whole care package. With an array of other professionals at the ambulance services disposal, the incidence of a patient being admitted to hospital should greatly be reduced. The ambulance service almost needs to be separated into two functions—that of dealing with life-threatening calls where the patient is rapidly transported to an acute hospital, and, secondly, dealing with primary care and wellbeing issues where joint working practices with local partners is essential.

Conclusions

There have previously been discussions which proposed that ambulance services should move away from the NHS and become part of the fire and rescue service (Knight 2013). There is, however, a very strong case which means that a modern ambulance service cannot be operated independently from the rest of the NHS.

The care of patients has to be integrated between agencies and hospitals. Removing the ambulance service away from the NHS could only serve to complicate and reduce interagency working. Whilst working closely with colleagues in the fire and rescue service and the police is essential at road traffic collisions and major incidents, these only represent a small percentage of the workload of an ambulance service. The need for improving relationships between the three blue services has been recognised and the Joint Emergency Services Interoperability Programme (JESIP) is underway, which was the key discussion issue in Chap. 9.

Paramedics are required to liaise with other healthcare professionals. It could be the doctor or nurse they are handing over to at a hospital or a patient's GP. It could be that the paramedic has to refer a patient to a mental health team, emergency nursing team or other community support organisation. In order for that paramedic to be respected amongst other allied professionals, the paramedic role needs to be understood and should come under the same NHS umbrella.

It is possible that by investing more into pre-hospital care, costs could be reduced later on. Admission into a hospital is extremely expensive and should always be avoided if feasible and possible. In order to achieve this, pre-hospital provision needs to evolve. By improving the assessment skills of paramedics and widening their treatment options, more people would be successfully managed in the community. This could go hand in hand with ambulance services being able to take more of a co-ordination role with other community health providers such as nursing and mental health teams. Combining the skills of some of these healthcare professionals could develop a technically less expensive workforce which is well placed to increase their community care roles.

Bibliography

Blyth, M. (2013). A primer on austerity, debt and morality plays. In *Austerity: The history of a dangerous idea* (p. 1). New York: Oxford University Press.

Campion, E.W., & Morrissey, S. (2013). A different model-medical care in Cuba. *The New England Journal of Medicine, 368*(4), 297–299.

Fitz, D. (2011). Why does health care in Cuba cost 96 % less than in the US? *Links International Journal of Socialist Renewal.* 5 Jan 2011.

Foster, J., Dale, J., & Jessopp, L. (2001). A qualitative study of older people's views of out-of-hours services. *British Journal of General Practice, 51*(1), 719–723.

House of Lords. (2012). Office of National Statistics. *Public service and demographic change committee.* p. 801.

Knight, K. (2013). *FACING THE FUTURE: Findings from the review of efficiencies and operations in fire and rescue authorities in England.* London: The Stationery Office.

Lilley, R. (2013). Fiddling while the NHS burns. *Fiddling while the NHS burns.* 12 July 2013.

Pilkington, P. (2013). Teleology and market equilibrium: Manifesto for a general theory of prices. *Fixing the Economists.* WordPress.com. Accessed 16 Aug 2013.

Robert Till started his ambulance career in 2000. Robert has worked as a paramedic, HEMS paramedic, Special Operations Response Team responder, duty manager within the Emergency Operations Centre and executive officer to the CEO of West Midlands Ambulance Service. He has represented West Midlands Ambulance Service at National Events and has pursued his interest in leadership and modernising ambulance services by working closely with Dr Marsh.

Dr Anthony Marsh QAM, SBStJ, DSci (Hon), MBA, MSc, FASI started his ambulance career in Essex in 1987. He relocated as the chief executive officer of the West Midlands Ambulance Service in 2006. Anthony holds a Master of Science degree in strategic leadership as well as a Master in Business Administration (MBA) and has been awarded a Doctorate from the University of Wolverhampton. In addition to his responsibilities as CEO he was appointed chair of the Association of Ambulance Chief Executives, lead for the National Ambulance Resilience Unit and is also the CEO of East of England Ambulance Service. Dr Marsh was awarded Queens Ambulance Service Medal in the 2014.

Part IV
Looking to the Future

Chapter 12
The Ambulance Service of the Future

Mark Docherty, Andrew Carson and Matthew Ward

Context and Background: The Case for Change

Around the world, services for urgent and emergency healthcare needs are becoming busier, and the risk is that the current configuration of services will become unsustainable in years to come if services do not change radically. There are a number of reasons why current demand is outstripping the supply of services:

- The demographics of the population are changing, with an increasingly elderly population living with complex health needs and multiple long-term conditions. This population is also responsible for a shift in most developed countries with regard to the demographic of major trauma that has historically been dominated by young adult males and which is now seeing a shift towards falls in over 65-year-olds being the main source of major trauma cases.
- A younger generation of consumerists, who are used to an internet world of immediate response, rising expectations and a desire to see services delivered in a more convenient way.
- We have a significant global recession, where funding for health care just will not keep up with demand that is delivered as 'more of the same'.
- There is a national shortfall in the workforce of nurses, general practitioners (GPs), hospital emergency department (ED) doctors, paramedics and a whole

M. Docherty (✉) · A. Carson · M. Ward
West Midlands Ambulance Service NHS Foundation Trust, Millennium Point,
Waterfront Way, Brierley Hill, Dudley, West Midlands DY5 1LX, UK
e-mail: mark@docherty.info

A. Carson
e-mail: Andrew.carson@wmas.nhs.uk

M. Ward
e-mail: matthew.ward@wmas.nhs.uk

© Springer International Publishing Switzerland 2015
P. Wankhade, K. Mackway-Jones (eds.), *Ambulance Services,*
DOI 10.1007/978-3-319-18642-9_12

range of other allied health professionals. Even if financial resources were not scarce, there simply is not the number of healthcare professionals available to deliver care in the same way going forward.

- We have a confused, urgent and emergency care system. There is an inconsistent way in which care is delivered in different settings. Accident and emergency departments are sometimes called EDs, but the care offered at each may differ. The range of services varies even more between different care settings that call themselves minor injury units (MIUs), and there is also an array of other services, such as immediate care centres, health centres, walk-in centres and many other terms that mean that the public simply get confused as to where they should go.
- People simply choose the place to go depending on what is easiest and provides the convenience that is desired. As a result of this, ambulance services and hospital EDs often become the default choice as these services are available 24 h a day, and they have therefore become a victim of their own success.

The National Health Services' (NHS) urgent and emergency care services provide life-saving care. The current system is under increasing pressure and NHS England wants to improve the urgent and emergency care system so patients get safe and effective care whenever they need it.

In January 2013, the NHS Medical Director Professor Sir Bruce Keogh announced a comprehensive review of the NHS urgent and emergency care system in England. A review of the implementation of the review's findings suggested that collaboration and integration were key themes in the system change and that there is no national one-size-fits-all approach.

The vision presented by the Keogh review is clear: For people with urgent needs that are not life-threatening, a local responsive service in the pre-hospital environment is a priority. Where people are found to have serious or life-threatening needs, then treatment in centralised centres with high expertise and good infrastructure will maximise good clinical outcomes. This vision is demonstrated visually (Fig. 12.1, cited in Keogh (2013)).

In the event of an unplanned care need, a person has two routes into care services; a nonemergency route via a national 111 call number connects a patient to a call taker who, via an algorithm, assesses the patient's health needs and signposts them to the most appropriate service for their needs locally or, if necessary, dispatches an ambulance for the person to have further assessment.

This strategy is also founded on five clinical priorities:

1. Giving people the skills and confidence to self-care
2. Ensuring that people get the right care in the right place first time
3. Ensuring that appropriate services are available for people to use outside of hospital
4. Connecting urgent and emergency services together and ensuring they work as a system rather than different parts
5. Where people need specialist emergency care, ensuring this is provided in centres that have the right expertise and equipment

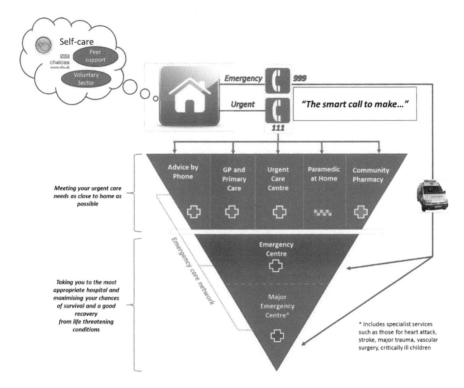

Fig. 12.1 The proposed look and design of the new system. (Keogh Review 2013, p. 23)

The Keogh review (2013) identified that:

> By extending paramedic training and skills, and supporting them with GPs and specialists, we will develop our 999 ambulances into mobile urgent treatment services capable of dealing with more people at scene, and avoiding unnecessary journeys to hospital.

In 2014–2015, England saw the number of emergency ambulance 999 calls reach ten million, meaning that a person will call 999 on average every 5 or 6 years, so it is unlikely that we will ever be in a position to educate the public properly about how to use an ambulance service. What we need to design is a service that can respond appropriately to a person's request for assistance irrespective of the need. This means that in future, ambulance services will need a greater repertoire of response models that are either provided or available to ambulance staff.

Specialist Centres for Emergency Care

Local general hospitals have traditionally offered a range of diagnostic and treatment options for most conditions, but increasingly some services are being concentrated in more specialised centres. The treatment for a heart attack, for example has changed from 40 years ago, when bed rest was the treatment of choice (with a 25 % in hospital mortality) to the modern treatment of mechanically unblocking the coronary artery, which produces a much better clinical outcome and reduced mortality. Major traumas, hyper-acute stroke services and vascular and neonatal services are other examples of services that have gone or are undergoing reconfiguration.

Increasingly, therefore, we will see more services developed in specialist emergency centres, which will be fewer in number, and therefore ambulance clinicians will be required to deliver a wider cadre of skills, including diagnostic and treatment to ensure that patients are taken to the centre that can most effectively deal with the condition that the patient presents with (Berwick 2013).

The implications of this must continue to be approached at the level of the whole health economy, with intelligent commissioning decisions being taken to focus on the best outcomes for patients through appropriate alternative care pathways that are underpinned by a clear infrastructure of primary care services, including GP services, walk-in centres, MIUs, district nursing services and well-established links with social care. All of this needs to be available 7 days a week to support the higher level urgent and emergency services, such as EDs, to avoid the latter being overwhelmed by conditions that could be managed more simply in a setting more local and more clinically appropriate to the patient.

Implications for Ambulance Services

Ambulance services are in the front line of this rising tide of urgent and emergency care activity and ambulance clinicians find themselves acting as gatekeepers to pathways that are most appropriate for the patient in front of them. Commissioners have tended to focus on the importance of reducing conveyance rates to EDs, but this has not always been matched by the funding required to support the development of alternative pathways that improve the outcome for patients. If patient safety, clinical effectiveness and patient experience are to guide the direction of travel for commissioners and the wider health economy, then the focus must be on *safer care, closer to home* and a realisation for clinicians and patients that *home is normal*. Simply concentrating on reducing conveyance rates carries the potential to create huge risks for patients from a clinical perspective.

A further issue for the ambulance sector is that the traditional training for paramedics and other frontline clinicians has been to take the well-established airway, breathing and circulation (ABC) approach as the basis for their clinical assessment. As ambulance trusts move into the new world of assessing patients and accessing newly developed patient pathways via the developing infrastructure of more appropriate local services, they will need to develop the skills to undertake a rapid, safe and effective assessment, once they have assured themselves that a patient does not need to be conveyed urgently to an emergency care facility (National Audit Office 2010). This might take the form of a more traditional medical model approach to history taking and systemic examination or another alternative would be the paramedic pathfinder, a model based on the Manchester Triage Tool and adapted as a series of algorithms to enable a rapid face-to-face assessment of a patient, aiding the decision of which alternative pathway to use. The importance with the paramedic pathfinder approach is the need for this to be supported by the infrastructure of more local services as alternatives to the ED. The inevitable effect of a more involved face-to-face patient assessment is the potential impact for:

- Increasing on-scene times and, therefore, overall job-cycle times, reducing logistical efficiency and the impact on time measures performance standards
- Increased requirement for clinical supervision in order to support the widening of the scope of practice being required by ambulance clinicians
- Increasing the amount of equipment for diagnosis and treatment required
- Increasing the requirement for drugs and the management and legislation surrounding prescribers and nonprescribers

Clinical, human resource (HR) and operational colleagues will need to work together to minimise the potentially disruptive impact of these elements on a system already facing huge operational pressures.

The Digital Patient Record and Integration with the Wider Health Economy

In the UK, many ambulance trusts still use a paper Patient Report Form (PRF), whilst a recent nationally driven initiative to develop an electronic patient record is currently being wound up. New systems are currently being developed but there are a few key principles to be considered.

- A digital patient record should not attempt to be an electronic version of the PRF as this would miss huge opportunities for enhancing patient care.
- Frontline staff should be able to see clear advantages in the delivery of care to their patients' on-scene so that compliance with and use of the digital record is maximised.
- The system should include live recording of data from monitors, such as ECG, oximetry, capnography, temperature, etc. This will produce a far richer source of information for each patient that is live data, enabling far timelier reporting of clinical metrics to triangulate more meaningfully with operational, HR and finance metrics within the organisation.
- Information from previous contacts with the ambulance service should be available via the system, enabling pre-population of key fields such as past medical history, allergies and medication. This should save on-scene time.
- Every effort should be made to match the case to NHS number, bringing the ambulance services into line with the rest of the NHS in using this as the primary identifier for each patient. This will enable access to the summary care record, where available, giving up-to-date information about current medication, allergies and key diagnoses that can be compared with the historical record and giving further opportunities for reducing on-scene time. Another advantage of

using the NHS number would be the potential for accessing better outcome data for individual patients.

- Development teams should liaise with local initiatives in their areas that are currently working to produce shared health and social care records, giving the potential for access to patient care plans, details of key workers etc.
- Each face-to-face contact should result in an appropriate report to the patient's GP and other interested parties, such as safeguarding referrals, referrals to community diabetic teams, etc., thus enabling easy identification of higher volume service users by GPs, as well as reducing the time taken on-scene to make direct referrals by telephone.
- The system should be able to link with hospital patient administration systems (PAS) for pre-alerting; possibly generating SMS texts to primary percutaneous coronary intervention (PPCI) teams so that ST-elevation myocardial infarction (STEMI) patients, for example can be conveyed directly to the PPCI suite or Face Arm Speech Test (FAST)-positive stroke patients could be conveyed directly to CT.
- Systems with video capability could, with clear policies around maintenance of confidentiality, be used to stream images to the trauma desk for specialist advice, stream video to secondary care colleagues to bring consultants into the home remotely for advice around the need to convey or use of alternative pathways.
- A video function could also allow crews to contribute remotely to morbidity and mortality meetings for cases that they have been involved in, enhancing their own personal development.
- Consistent coding is of the utmost importance when considering benchmarking, both within the organization and comparing with historical performance, as well as comparing with other trusts. A well-recognized coding system, such as SNOMED CT®, should be used and code sets should be agreed nationally, with data entry streamlined through appropriate use of templates. Rapid assessment using the Paramedic Pathfinder or Medical Model could be adapted for data to be entered via templates. Data entry should be flexible, so that patient care is not interfered with but there should be an ability to complete data entry after handover.
- Consistent coding should enable more detailed analysis of clinical performance in individual cases, as well as groups of cases such as STEMI patients, diabetic hypos etc. Audit departments should have good reporting systems to provide timely information to the board level for triangulation with other metrics in the organisation.
- Individual clinicians should be able to review their cases for reflective practice, enhancing opportunities for personal development, as well as comparison with peers (clearly this would need to be done in a nonthreatening way to avoid any negative impact on individual clinicians).

- The system should link to other resources, such as British National Formulary (BNF), TOXBASE®, Directory of Services, UK Ambulance Service Clinical and Practice Guidelines, enabling crews to access relevant information rapidly with regard to the patient they are treating. Links to prescribing software such as BNF should promote safer treatment by paramedics on-scene, reducing the risk of allergic reactions or drug interactions.
- With the current trend towards far more patient-focused care, post Francis report and Berwick review, software packages are currently under development for use by patients themselves (e.g. Health Fabric) that enable patients to link to their GP and hospital records, as well as helping patients to develop their own personalized care plans. If ambulance systems are to be future proofed, then they should be able to link in with these packages as well, where patients allow, so that a patient's own views can be seen and taken into consideration. This, along with telemetry and remote monitoring of high-risk patients, will mean the ambulance service will have a role in preventative and anticipatory urgent and emergency care.

Conclusion

With the rising tide of activity levels, changing demographics, service reconfigurations and changing patterns of urgent and emergency care provision, it is vital that a health economy-wide approach is adopted by all parties to develop clear patient pathways locally. The focus for ambulance trusts must be safer care, closer to home and not merely reducing conveyance rates (House of Commons Health Committee 2013; Keogh Report 2013). This will involve intelligent commissioning and collaboration between health and social care across the entire health economy. Simply doing much more of the same is not a long-term solution and often has a direct impact on issues such as the delivery of mandatory training and personal development reviews, which are key features that underpin any sustainable change within any modern, learning organization.

Such change within ambulance trusts can only be achieved through good communication across all directorates at board level, with a recognition that everyone is working towards the same goal of providing the best possible care to every patient having contact with the service. In addition to good internal communication across all directorates and throughout all levels of the organization, from board to front line and back, effective communication must be fostered between partner health and social care organizations across the health economy. The digital patient record and integration with the wider NHS is likely to be one of the most crucial cultural developments for the future.

References

Berwick, D. (2013). *A promise to learn—A commitment to act: improving the safety of patients in England*. London: Department of Health.

House of Commons Health Committee. (2013). *Urgent and emergency services second report of session 2013–2014*. London: The Stationery Office Limited.

Keogh, B. (2013). *Transforming urgent and emergency care services in England. Urgent and emergency care review, end of phase 1 report*. London: NHS England.

National Audit Office. (2010). *Major trauma care in England*. London: The Stationery Office.

Mark Docherty is the director of Nursing, Quality and Clinical Commissioning for West Midlands Ambulance Service NHS Foundation Trust. West Midlands Ambulance Service NHS Foundation Trust serves a population of 5.36 million people covering an area of more than 5000 square miles in the heart of England, and as the region's emergency ambulance service responds to around 3000 '999' calls each day. Mark has previously been the ambulance commissioner for London Ambulance Service, and in 2013 gave evidence to the House of Commons Health Committee on urgent care that led to the Urgent and Emergency Services Second Report (2013).

Dr Andrew Carson is the Medical Director for West Midlands Ambulance Service NHS Foundation Trust. Dr Carson has been a General Practitioner (GP) at a Medical Centre in Birmingham UK for 26 years. He is also an Associate Dean for GP Training for the Workforce Deanery in the West Midlands where he has been heavily involved in the training of GPs for around 15 years. He has also been a Clinical Director for an Urgent Care Centre. Dr Carson is a Fellow of the Royal College of General Practitioners and has a strong track record for innovative and strategic thinking. He has been involved in a number of research projects that have resulted in papers being published in the medical press.

Matthew Ward is a consultant paramedic working for West Midlands Ambulance Service NHS Foundation Trust. Matt has been a paramedic for 15 years, and specialises in emergency care. He was the head of Cardiac and Stroke Management for West Midlands Ambulance Service NHS Foundation Trust and was responsible for implementing a number of successful changes to clinical guidelines and pathways for cardiac, stroke and resuscitation care. He chaired the NHS Midlands and East Stroke Review during which he lead on the modelling of the new Hyper Acute Stroke Units and more recently also chaired the Birmingham and Black Country Stroke Review.

Chapter 13
Future Perspectives for the UK Ambulance Services: Evolution Rather than Revolution

Kevin Mackway-Jones and Paresh Wankhade

Context and Background

Ambulance services will always be needed or will they? It is easy to assume that just because many services are overwhelmed by current demand, they will grow and be present forever. However, what we have now has often arisen organically, and it just does not follow that the form that has evolved over past time has the right physical assets, capability and functionality to survive in the future. Several chapters in this book, notably those by Williams, Newton and Harris, Docherty and Carson, Jormakka and Lambert and others, also offer perspectives on the future of the prehospital care that raise important issues about the nature of the ambulance work and the changing societal–cultural context. We do not intend to add further complexity to these debates, but aim to essay an overview of these issues which of course do not all point unequivocally in the same direction. In the face of an apparently emerging consensus among academics and experts, it is worth pointing out that many contentious themes still resonate and are not resolved. They primarily concern with the 3Ss—issues of structures, skills and science.

So are there any fixed points around which we can imagine what might make a future ambulance service? Are there any medical or social conditions that can defy the desired move to community care? Are there any diagnostics or treatments that will require the patient to be moved whatever the political and economic imperatives? Are there any patients whose emergency health needs will require an immediate response? The answer to all these questions is, of course, maybe.

K. Mackway-Jones (✉)
North West Ambulance Service NHS Trust, Ladybridge Hall, Chorley New Road,
Heaton, BL1 5DD Bolton, UK
e-mail: kevin.Mackway-Jones@nwas.nhs.uk

P. Wankhade
Edge Hill Business School, Edge Hill University, Room B204, Ormskirk L39 4QP, UK
e-mail: Paresh.Wankhade@edgehill.ac.uk

© Springer International Publishing Switzerland 2015
P. Wankhade, K. Mackway-Jones (eds.), *Ambulance Services,*
DOI 10.1007/978-3-319-18642-9_13

Let us take each question individually. What 'fixed points' might there be? The ambulance service is named around its vehicles—in particular, the vehicles used to transport patients. Does that mean that a service that does not have vehicles to move patients is no longer an ambulance service? Perhaps this is true in a historic sense but modern ambulance services have already evolved so as not to transport everyone that calls and no one is suggesting that they have lost their way (Lowthian et al. 2011). This change could conceivably continue such that in time, it might be the dispatch and arrival of the mobile health professional in an urgent of emergency situation that defines the ambulance function rather than the actual transport of the patient. This will, of course, require a change in the capability of the ambulance clinician and could even mean that healthcare professionals other than paramedics are best suited for the task. This argument debunks the idea that ambulance services are defined by the paramedics that work for them; paramedics are merely the pre-hospital clinicians that have evolved to work in the current service. The profession may not survive the natural selection required for the next step even if supported by appropriate decision support tools (Newton et al. 2014). Some of this, it can be argued, is linked to historical and legacy issues (Palmer 1983; Tangherlini 1998) and is about the evolution of the ambulance services primarily from a call-handling and transportation service, incorporating some aspects of patient care with an increasingly wider role as an outlet to other National Health Services (NHSs) and in ensuring that patients can access the facilities closer to their home (Department of Health (DH) 2005; DH 2010; National Audit Office (NAO) 2011).

So are there any conditions that are not amenable to community care? Probably not in a system without economic constraints. After all, everything *can* be provided at home or in mobile units in the community, even surgery and intensive care if money is no object. But we do not work (and are never likely to work) in such a system, so financial reality dictates that the economies of scale and concentration of skills that we currently call hospitals are likely to survive albeit in reduced numbers. Does this, then, give us a clue about a future ambulance service configuration? Well yes, it seems likely that there will always be a need for patients to be moved from home and community care to specialist hospital care, and it further seems likely that some of these patients will need more than unaccompanied transport. This is ambulance care.

Over and above this are there any diagnostics or treatments that will require the patient to be moved? Again in a system with limitless resources, it might always be possible to move the equipment to the patient but this seems unlikely to be a real option. Thus, patients will have to move and, again, some may require health service professional support while doing so. This does not necessarily mean that ambulances will be used, as other means of transport could be deployed, nor does it necessarily mean that ambulance professionals will be involved as other health professionals could deliver the service; but whatever it is called, it is ambulance care in all but name. Williams in his chapter makes a similar point about the need for an honest and open debate about the future of the ambulance services, so that the correct education, skill sets, operational models and functionality can be identified for the next decade.

Finally, are there any patents whose emergency health needs will require an immediate response? Some would argue that all emergencies are a failure of prevention, protection and planning and that all accidents are the result of failure to mitigate recognisable risk (the latter being the reason that, in the UK, Accident and Emergency Departments are changing their names to Emergency Departments) but others would merely reply that everyone eventually dies and some will die unexpectedly and without a plan in place; this is the point of emergency. It seems likely that some form of reactive service able to respond immediately to the perception of a health emergency will always be required. This function is of course currently provided by the ambulance service. However, saving lives can no longer be regarded as other than one priority among many responsibilities by an emergency practitioner, and the pace of reform is a growing international concern (Heightman and McCallion 2011). Other recent publications such as the NHS Confederation Urgent and Emergency Care Forum's "Ripping Off the Sticking Plaster" (NHS Confederation 2014) and the Paramedic Evidence-Based Education Project (PEEP) report on paramedic education and training (Lovegrove and Davis 2013) highlight various organisational and cultural challenges facing ambulance services in meeting increasingly complex forms of patient demand.

So what does the future actually hold? No one knows for sure but it seems likely that the health needs of the population and the configuration of health services will always require two functions currently provided by ambulance services. First, a means of supported transport of patients in the community to services provided in healthcare facilities; second, a responsive, professional, timely outreaching emergency diagnosis and management service. These are the core of current ambulance services and will be the core of any future service. What will change is the means of delivery and the professional that delivers the service. Technology will enable better remote triage; increasingly skilled practitioners will use better decision support mechanisms to deliver more sophisticated healthcare and vehicle design will evolve in ways yet to be imagined.

There is a significant body of literature suggesting opportunities for the ambulance services to help reduce unplanned hospital admissions through treating or referring at scene or via telephone rather than transportation to hospitals (Cooper et al. 2007; Halter et al. 2010; Mason et al. 2007; Woollard 2007; Gray and Walker 2008). Shifting the emergency care model in this direction was a central feature of the 'Taking Healthcare to the Patient' report (DH 2005) and the Keogh Urgent and Emergency Care Review suggested to develop ambulances into 'mobile urgent treatment services' (NHS England 2013, p. 8). A lot of progress has been made on these aspects in the past decade or so. There is a developed programme and progression route for paramedic education in the country now. Many of the ambulance trusts in England now deploy trained 'consultant/critical care paramedics' who now triage the calls in the control room to 'hear and treat' the patients, thus saving unnecessary ambulance journeys or patient transportation to the hospital Emergency Department. Better vehicles and use of technology to better the science are also on agenda. The Helen Hamlyn Centre for Design's partnership with the Vehicle Design Department at the Royal College of Art, Imperial College Healthcare NHS Trust and the London Ambulance Service to develop modern day ambulances is another example of the developing technology (Fusari and Muhammed 2011).

Newton and Harris in their piece argue that any doctrine for reform must be coupled with a clear concept of operation which is likely to see the traditional transport function progressively replaced by a more skilled and educated paramedic profession, capable of delivering critical decision-making, managing and treating increasing numbers of patients presenting with urgent primary care and emergency conditions, thus making the paramedic more relevant to present and future patient populations (Newton and Hodge 2012). As Middleton says, 'only when ambulance systems are joined to health services, providing the prehospital phase of emergency care, with paramedics assessing patients in a structured, risk-aware form based in clinical reasoning, and with processes, systems and interventions based on proven effectiveness measured by clinical outcome at later stages in the patient journey, will Australian ambulance services truly have come into the twenty-first century'. This is so very true for us in the UK as well.

To conclude, ambulance services are not solely a health construct but also they exist in society and reflect its' culture. It is easy to take the present and imagine it as set in stone but of course it is not. Whatever changes do come about one thing is for sure— that they will not be uniform. One size definitely will not fit all. We would be willing to bet, however, that whatever the outcome of the continued refinement and evolution we will see recognisable ambulances (by whatever name) crewed by paramedical professionals (by whatever name) delivering ambulance services (by whatever name) well into the future. As Alex Pollock's chapter on the history of the ambulance service in this volume shows—evolution, not revolution, is the way.

References

Cooper, S., O'Carroll, J., Jenkin, A., & Badger, B. (2007). Collaborative practices in unscheduled emergency care: role and impact of the emergency care practitioner—qualitative and summative findings. *Emergency Medicine Journal, 24,* 625–629.

DH. (2005). *Taking healthcare to the patient: Transforming NHS ambulance services.* London: Department of Health.

DH. (2010). *Building the evidence base in pre-hospital urgent and emergency care: A review of research evidence and priorities for future research.* London: Department of Health.

Fusari, G., & Muhammed. (2011). Redesigning the ambulance: Improving mobile emergency healthcare. The Helen Hamlyn Centre for Design, The Royal College of Art, London.

Gray, J. T., & Walker, A. (2008). Avoiding admissions from the ambulance service: a review of elderly patients with falls and patients with breathing difficulties seen by emergency care practitioners in South Yorkshire. *Emergency Medicine Journal, 25,* 168–171.

Halter, M., Vernon, S., Snooks, H., Porter, A., Close, J., Moore, F., et al. (2010). Complexity of the decision-making process of ambulance staff for assessment and referral of older people who have fallen: A qualitative study. *Emergency Medicine Journal, 28,* 44–45.

Heightman, A. J. and McCallion, T. (2011). Management lessons from Pinnacle: Key messages given to EMS leaders at the 2011 conference. *Journal of Emergency Medical Services, 36*(10), 50–54.

Lovegrove, M., & Davis, J., (2013). *Maximising paramedics' contribution to the delivery of high quality and cost effective patient care.* High Wycombe: Buckinghamshire New University.

Lowthian, J. A., Cameron, P. A., Stoelwinder, J. U., Curtis, A., Currell, A., Cooke, M. W., et al. (2011). Increasing utilisation of emergency ambulances. *Australian Health Review, 35,* 63–69.

Mason, S., Knowles, E., Colwell, B., Dixon, S., Wardrope, J., Gorringe, R., et al. (2007). Effectiveness of paramedic practitioners in attending 999 calls from elderly people in the community: Cluster randomised controlled trial'. *British Medical Journal, 335,* 919–925.

NHS Confederation. (2014). *Ripping off the sticking plaster: Whole-systems solutions for urgent and emergency care.* London: NHS Confederation.

NHS England. (2013). *Transforming urgent and emergency care in England: Urgent and emergency care review. Phase 1 report.* Leeds: NHS England.

National Audit Office (NAO). (2011). *Transforming NHS ambulance services.* London: TSO.

Newton, A., & Hodge, D. (2012). The ambulance service: The past, present and future'. *Journal of Paramedic Practice, 4*(5), 303–305.

Newton, M., Tunn, E., Moses, I., Ratcliffe, D., & Mackway-Jones, K. (2014). Clinical navigation for beginners: The clinical utility and safety of the paramedic pathfinder. *Emergency Medicine Journal,* e29–34. doi:10.1136/emermed-2012-202033.

Palmer, C. E. (1983). Trauma junkies and street work: Occupational behavior of paramedics and emergency medical technicians. *Journal of Contemporary Ethnography, 12*(2), 162–183.

Tangherlini, T. (1998). *Talking trauma: A candid look at paramedics through their tradition of tale-telling.* Mississippi: University Press of Mississippi.

Woollard, M. (2007). Paramedic practitioners and emergency admissions. *British Medcial Journal, 335,* 893–894.

Prof. Kevin Mackway-Jones was appointed as a consultant at the Manchester Royal Infirmary in 1993 and became a professor in the year 2001. He has published widely on the practice and theory of Emergency Medicine, both books (*Advanced Paediatric Life Support, Major Incident Medical Management and Support, Emergency Triage* amongst others) and academic papers. His main research interests are diagnostic strategies, psychosocial care and major incident management. Apart from consulting at the Manchester Royal Infirmary and the Royal Manchester Children's Hospital, he is also an executive medical director at the North West Ambulance Service, civilian consultant advisor to the British Army and head of the North Western School of Emergency Medicine. He is the webmaster for www.bestbets.org and the St Emlyn's Virtual Hospital through which he runs an MSc in Emergency Medicine. He was an editor in chief of the *Emergency Medicine Journal* from 2005–2013.

Prof. Paresh Wankhade is a Professor of Leadership and Management at the Edge Hill University Business School. He has done his PhD in Ambulance Performance & Culture Change Management from the University of Liverpool, UK. He is the founder editor of the *International Journal of Emergency Services* (an Emerald group Publication) and is recognised as an expert in the field of emergency management. He has chaired special tracks on leadership and management of emergency services at major international conferences including the annual European Academy of Management (EURAM) Conference, British Academy of Management Conference and Public Administration Committee (PAC) Conference. His research and publications focus on analyses of strategic leadership, organisational culture, organisational change and interoperability within the emergency services. His publications have contributed to inform debates around interoperability of public services and challenges faced by individual organisations. His latest book on *Social Capital, Sociability and Community Development* explores these issues including the state of the pre-hospital care in eight selected case study countries (UK, USA, China, India, Bangladesh, Japan, Netherlands and South Africa) around the world.

Chapter 14
International Perspectives: Australian Ambulance Services in 2020

Paul M Middleton

Introduction

Australia is huge, with a landmass similar to North America, but with only 27 million citizens, compared to over 350 million in the USA. Western Australia (WA) is the third largest subdivision of a country in the world; it is, at over 2.5 million square kilometres, larger than Alaska, the largest US state, and is only superseded by the northern region of Brazil and the Sakha Republic of Russia. Ambulance services in Australia are disparate in all dimensions, using varying combinations of personnel, including community first responders, volunteer ambulance crews, paramedics, extended care paramedic (ECP) services, air ambulance and rescue. Although Australian states and territories are responsible for the provision of ambulance services, WA and the Northern Territory contract non-government bodies such as St. John Ambulance to provide patient care and transport with all ancillary facilities. Australian ambulance services are funded largely by a combination of direct State or Territory revenue, subscription schemes and user charges. The total 2006/2007 revenue for ambulance services across Australia was $ 1.6 billion, with government providing 64.8% of the total allocation (New South Wales Department of Health 2008).

P. M. Middleton (✉)
Discipline of Emergency Medicine, University of Sydney / DREAM Collaboration, Sydney,
52 Kempbridge Avenue, Seaforth, NSW 2092, Australia
e-mail: pmmiddleton@gmail.com

© Springer International Publishing Switzerland 2015
P. Wankhade, K. Mackway-Jones (eds.), *Ambulance Services,*
DOI 10.1007/978-3-319-18642-9_14

State of Australian Ambulance Services

Paramedics in Australia are not regulated at a state, territory or federal level, and the issue of registration incites impassioned arguments. Accreditation of paramedic continuing education and competence to practice is currently solely managed by individual ambulance services, albeit in association with voluntary continuing professional development (CPD) schemes run by representative bodies. A recent poll of paramedics by Paramedics Australasia attracted 4000 responses, with 86.7% supporting registration under a national scheme (Bange and van Biljon 2012).The implications of this lack of registration are that there are no validated and independent measures of knowledge or competence transferable between services, states or even countries, and there are no common curricula or definitions accepted by employers (Thom et al. 2014). Another significant handicap arising from the lack of registration is that the opportunity to self-regulate and maintain standards of practice, the hallmark of any professional group, is denied to paramedics as a group, and therefore, this remains a function of employers. Maintenance of standards and disciplining of poor performers usually then become an adversarial battle between employers, paramedics and union representatives.

Paramedics in Australia also perform much of their work according to either protocols or guidelines (Shaban et al. 2004). Being a specific set of step-by-step instructions to perform a defined task, protocols carry the implication that their content has to be adhered to with no room for choice and judgement, whereas guidelines suggest that there is room to interpret the instructions in the light of patient condition and available evidence. Clinical guidelines should be based on the best available evidence and provide recommendations for practice about specific clinical interventions for specific patient populations; however, it is uncertain whether either protocols or guidelines which drive paramedic practice are based on appropriate methodology or whether they solely reflect eminence-based opinion. Furthermore, and most importantly, paramedics are not taught to work within any diagnostic paradigm. There has been much contemplation regarding medical diagnosis, whether using exhaustive, hypothetico-deductive or pattern-recognition techniques; however, this has not translated in Australia to a similar discussion within paramedicine.

Paramedics in Australia largely concentrate on the traditional delivery of prehospital care. This means that prioritisation is carried out on 000 call receipt, in many jurisdictions using dedicated software, such as the ProQA®/Medical Priority Dispatch System (MPDS)®, using the chief complaint and a set of predetermined questions. On arrival at scene, Australian paramedics carry out patient assessment with variable degrees of systematic structure, not always orientated around the identification of threat to life or the potential for deterioration, and sometimes having more in common with the comprehensive secondary survey than the risk-identifying primary survey.

Coupled with a slow incremental increase in the perceived importance of identifying early abnormalities in physiology in order to risk-stratify patients, and a lack of focus in targeted history taking, barriers to the effective identification of at-risk patients, and to the ability of paramedics and ambulance services to perform a valid secondary triage of patients on scene are significant. As a consequence, paramedics are not trained in the effective assessment of risk and the potential for deterioration, and thus inappropriate non-transport decisions may be made. Without the ability to recognise sentinel symptoms and signs and to place these in the context of the patient's physiological condition, errors occur in advice given to patients and in the weight placed on history and examination (Middleton and Malone 2010).

Issues have been identified with both maintenance and supervision of quality of care in the prehospital phase of emergency care. Callaham (1997) stated that '… because there is such a paucity of scientific support for EMS interventions and because monitoring of outcomes and adverse effects is so poor, a serious re-examination of EMS practice is indicated'. This is especially relevant in Australia, as there exist a number of highly technologically advanced ambulance services, allowing a large number of clinical interventions, but serving a vast area with a sparse population. This leads to infrequent performance of many interventions, with frequency often being in inverse proportion to the urgency of the situation.

Experimental projects in Australia have trialled extended care models of paramedicine, enabling ambulance services to elect not to transport patients to hospital, in instances where the chief complaint is one which can be managed with either extended role paramedic skills or through alternate referral patterns (Blacker et al. 2009). This appears to have been effective in many jurisdictions, based upon metrics such as a reduction in the number of patients transferred to emergency departments (ED); however, there has been little other measurement of effectiveness as evaluation has largely been confined to assessment of structure and process, rather than patient outcome. This satisfies the need for services to be seen to be working to reduce the emergency care burden but does not allow recognition of any true value to patients.

The final, and potentially the most important aspect of all, is that only in WA is data from the prehospital phase of care linked to date from in-hospital care, to allow investigation of outcomes in patients treated and transported by ambulance services. In all other jurisdictions, data generated within ambulance, comprising automated dispatch data and increasingly, electronically captured patient healthcare details, including patient history, examination findings, physiological variables and both pharmacological and physical interventions, are entirely separate from data gathered within the ED or hospital. Data transfer from ambulance to hospital is largely printed-paper-based even when a prehospital electronic healthcare record is used, negating many potential benefits of timely information sharing. There is also minimal return and sharing of hospital process and outcome data with ambulance services, leading to the situation where the majority of services and paramedics have no idea of patient outcome, beyond a very limited number of patients included in quality registries such as those with severe trauma. The lack of this knowledge means that there is no way to judge the effectiveness of the entire prehospital phase of care, whether on a system or individual patient level (Al-Harbi et al. 2012; Dean et al. 2001).

Australian Ambulance Services in 2020

This section highlights few key focus areas that would help to revolutionise the paramedicine and prehospital care in the next decades. Each of the areas is discussed in some detail.

Ambulance Services as the Prehospital Element of the Health Service

The first and most critical step is the philosophical conversion of Australian ambulance services from separate and disparate emergency services to fundamental elements of the health services, acknowledging that they provide the prehospital phase of emergency medical care. There is an almost irrefutable argument that, as the pathology which brings patients into the emergency care system is frequently undifferentiated and time-dependent, the processes of structured assessment, resuscitation, stabilisation and diagnosis should be taken to the patient to as great an extent as possible (Brun et al. 2014; Ebinger et al. 2014a, b).

The implementation of such a philosophical paradigm across Australia will be most effectively organised and driven by a central, federal agenda, which in itself will need to be driven by the processes and practices of the clinical quality movement. Australia has a federal agency responsible for clinical quality, The Australian Commission on Safety and Quality in Health Care (2014) created by Health Ministers in 2006 and funded by all governments on a cost-sharing basis, to lead and coordinate healthcare safety and quality improvements in Australia (Australian Commission on Safety and Quality in Health Care, Governance 2014). This is supported by organisations such as The Australian Institute for Health and Welfare, a national agency set up to provide information and statistics on Australia's health. Collaboration with the Council of Ambulance Authorities, the informal body formed to provide leadership for the provision of ambulance services in Australia, and having representatives from both ambulance executives and clinicians, is likely to be of significant importance.

Paramedic Registration

This description of ambulance services with an evolved place in the health system naturally lead to the next most important strategic step by 2020, which is national registration for paramedics. In their submission to the Australian Health Ministers' Advisory Council on options for regulation of paramedics, Paramedics Australasia identified a list of risks of paramedic practice in its current form, and seven areas that would benefit from registration (Table 14.1; Paramedics Australasia 2012).

Table 14.1 Risks and benefits in relation to paramedic registration. (Paramedics Australasia 2012)

Risks in paramedic practice	Benefits of registration
Invasive procedures	An independent complaints mechanism
Administration of scheduled drugs	Approved educational and practitioner standards to use the title 'paramedic'
Working away from supervision	Prevention of paramedics with 'issues' moving from job to job
Provision of complex and critical clinical assessments and care	Checks a condition of practice
Working in dangerous and uncontrolled settings	Compulsory and independent accreditation of training and education

Registration has a major impact in two specific areas—maintenance of education and practice quality, and self-regulation. As detailed in the Paramedics Australasia submission, compulsory, independent accreditation of both training and educational standards allows the development of a common curriculum for all paramedics, in both undergraduate and postgraduate settings. Registration can therefore clearly have benefits for paramedics, ambulance services and patients, ensuring high-quality education and practice, and would support moves toward integration within health services. Registration is potentially the single most important early step for ambulance services and government agencies to undertake for the future.

E-learning and the Education Revolution

The 'tyranny of distance' was mentioned earlier in the context of learning and continuing education in Australia. Currently, in 2014, there is a National Broadband Network being constructed across Australia, and although subject to infrastructural change driven by the prevailing political cycle, seems likely to deliver substantial capability in internet delivery. Australia's current internet download speed ranks 32nd in the world, at 5.8 Mbit/s, compared to the UK and the USA with almost twice this speed and is almost a quarter of the world leader, South Korea, with 22 Mbit/s (Australian Government Department of Communication 2012).

Notwithstanding this change, the ability of such a network to enable high-quality e-learning to distant sites, resulting in the implementation of asymmetric initiatives such as blended learning, combining online theory and face-to-face skills training; 'flipped classroom' models, with paramedics collaborating online then being guided through exercises in the classroom; and live discussion and guided learning through webinars, means that paramedic education is likely to be revolutionised. Implementing and utilising these technological innovations in the context of a national curriculum and supervised quality maintenance and CPD programs seem likely to exponentially increase these benefits.

Clinical Reasoning

Another radical but necessary evolution in Australian paramedicine, in order to deliver truly twenty-first century services integrated into the health system, is the development of a curriculum based on clinical reasoning. Linn defined this as 'the cognitive process that underlies diagnosis and management of a patient's presenting problem' and although potentially providing an educational challenge, is an absolute necessity to reduce risk for patients and allow paramedics to evolve into a discipline that is able to fit into the health service model as the initial element of emergency care (Linn et al. 2012).

Currently, as mentioned above, paramedics perform their function by following protocols, or at best less restrictive guidelines, in order to establish a presenting pattern of pathology that may be treated within a particular protocol. This methodology of practice carries with it, however, several inherent problems. Firstly, paramedics often contort presenting complaints into a 'diagnostic box', as they are told that they are unable to diagnose but may simply 'assess' a patient; they make the diagnosis fit the protocol. This clearly predisposes a patient to inappropriate or inadequate management, or both (Shaban et al. 2004; O'Hara et al. 2015).

Secondly, there is little structured risk assessment performed within the paramedic approach; therefore, delineation of the impact of pathology, degree of compensation, patient deterioration and prioritisation of interventions are limited to a substantial and worrying degree. Although many services and paramedic educators teach an advanced life support (ALS)/advanced trauma life support primary survey algorithm, the necessary theoretical underpinning is often absent to some extent, leading to a lack of appreciation not only of the value of measured physiological variables but also of the relative importance of abnormalities. Thus, for instance, a common error is the reliance on a normal oxygen saturation and systolic blood pressure to reassure paramedics that the patient is stable, whilst ignoring the presence of marked tachypnoea and tachycardia, which indicate deterioration but ongoing compensation and unlike the prior measures which, when abnormal, imply late loss of compensation (Cretikos et al. 2008).

Finally, rigid and linear assessment protocols, without the training and theoretical knowledge to estimate risk and consider underlying pathological processes, ensure that paramedics are seldom in a position to appreciate the potential for deterioration rather than actual deterioration which can be seen in front of them. The possibility of incipient airway obstruction, respiratory failure or decreasing perfusion and shock may take second place to obvious, but less serious, problems which may be stable such as limb injuries.

Clinical reasoning allows the presentation of more than one initial hypothesis, then the use of available information and structured questioning to reprioritise likely explanatory variables, using relative positive and negative findings to refine the likely diagnosis and prioritise interventions. A syllabus in clinical reasoning, even though not necessarily as comprehensive as that delivered within the context of a medical degree and postgraduate training, will still equip paramedics to consider the relative impact of disease, as well as to examine patients in relation to the potential for life threat, assign levels of risk and intervene without diagnosis. A clear outcome of the informed clinical reasoning approach is that there may then be a decreasing reliance on rigid protocols to determine paramedic practice and an increasing ability to use interventions based in clinical risk. In this way, the response to an emergency call may, in reality, constitute a genuine first point of contact with emergency care rather than a service simply for the transport of patients.

Extended Care Paramedic Models

Many ambulance services have experimented with ECP models, which are based in the paradigm change from 'taking the patient to care' to 'taking care to the patient'(Blacker et al. 2009). ECP programs range in theoretical and philosophical underpinning from the performance of simple nonemergency interventions, such as the changing of urinary catheters, wound care and suturing and the administration of antibiotics for minor infections, to the performance of '…thorough medical examinations, risk assessment and development of patient management plans based on a predominantly medical model' (New South Wales Health: Ambulance Service of New South Wales 0000). Although this appears to represent an important development in the role of ambulance services and paramedics as part of the health system, there appears to be no attempt at analysing the impact of the ECP model on patient outcomes.

   In keeping with most system innovation developed within the context of the bureaucratic health service model, measures of success are centred on metrics process such as the decrease in patient transports to hospital, and whether staff and patients 'like' the innovation. This approach to system analysis unfortunately sidesteps the question of whether it is actually good for patients, and does not recognise the intrinsic scientific problem that patients may simply be lost to follow up and therefore will not figure in any form of audit. Given that paramedics do not currently perform any structured history or examination based in the identification of risk or deterioration, documentation of less than optimal outcomes is currently very unlikely. Future ECP programs will need to be based on a predefined and scientifically designed plan to assess the programs not only in terms of the effect on the patient but also of the associated health economic effects.

Human Factors and Error

Clinical governance was discussed earlier with respect to the benefits of registration, however there are other vital areas for consideration, in particular relating to the prevention or minimisation of error and adverse events, and to maintenance of clinical quality. There is increasing recognition that there are patterns of related contributory components within adverse patient events, with an average of 10 con-

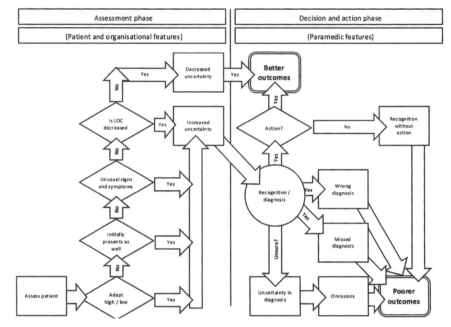

Fig. 14.1 Flow chart demonstrating possible relationships within some serious patient harm events (Price et al. 2013). *LOC* loss of consciousness

tributory factors per reported case (Price et al. 2013). This is particularly significant in prehospital care as resources, both human and technical, are extremely limited with little potential for escalation. Situations such as patient deterioration are magnified and exponentially worsened by coincident factors such as communication errors, case complexity, lack of room and adaptation from low to high acuity. Structured approaches may lend coherence and stratify risk and urgency in this situation, but the importance of recognising human factors within error is vital. Training in decision-making, largely based in realistic simulated scenarios, is likely to have a substantial impact on paramedics' ability to make good decisions in unfavourable and austere circumstances (Mundella et al. 2013; Fig. 14.1).

Cardiopulmonary Resuscitation Quality

The use of clinical governance in the maintenance of quality is similarly complex and far-reaching, but one area within which evidence is quickly accumulating to support change is in the measurement of interventional quality in emergency situations such as cardiac arrest. A worrying body of research has demonstrated that cardiopulmonary resuscitation (CPR) quality is highly variable in both prehospital and hospital-based environments and has shown wide variation in compression rates and depths, frequent long pauses in CPR, and hyperventilation during resuscitation care (Aufderheide et al. 2005; Wik et al. 2005; Milander et al. 1995). Conversely, intense focus on measuring and improving the quality of CPR has shown that direct measurement of these variables and the addition of real-time feedback drastically improves performance and patient outcomes such as survival (Abella 2013).

In light of the clear relationship between the quality of interventions such as CPR and improvement in patient outcomes, it is difficult to justify training or practice in the prehospital arena which is not subject to careful and continuous quality measurement and maintenance. This therefore needs to be a mandatory component of paramedic education and CPD. International jurisdictions such as King County in the USA have increased the survival from a 'shockable' cardiac arrest from 27% in 2002 to 62% in 2014 (Public Health, Seattle and King County 2014) in contrast to an average rate of approximately 20% in Australia, and an overall survival rate of 10% (Cheung et al. 2013) largely by the intensive measurement and improvement of CPR and system quality. Australian ambulance systems should adopt this approach as rapidly as possible.

Simulation

Given the previous discussion regarding the difficulties in education across large distances with staff and educators highly separated by geography, the use of simulation becomes inescapable. Clinical education has to incorporate the learning of scientific principles but also demands objective measures of competence in the domains of knowledge, skills, and behaviours (Rosen 2008). Practice is a fundamental component of learning and maintenance of skills in many disciplines and in particular in interventional clinical domains. Studies have shown that performance on ALS scenarios improved significantly with repetitive practice using a medical simulator compared to clinical experience alone (Wayne et al. 2010). Use of a computer-enhanced mannequin in a structured educational program, with opportunities for deliberate practice, yielded large, consistent and sustained improvements in residents' skills with little decay over time.

A recent systematic review and meta-analysis suggested that simulation was of particular benefit in learning and perfecting skill-based processes, with potentially improved effectiveness from 'booster' practice or 'spaced education', the inclusion of team and group dynamics, distraction and integrated feedback (Mundella et al. 2013). Research in emergency medicine residents also found simulation to be effective at teaching metacognitive strategies, or knowledge about when and how to use particular strategies for problem solving, an area particularly useful when attempting to educate paramedics in the techniques of managing undifferentiated patients under conditions of stress and multiple distractions (Bond et al. 2004). Future progression towards models of ambulance services integrated with health services is dependent on carefully planned educational strategies based on necessary outcomes.

Data

It was described earlier that ambulance data, albeit comprehensive, are not linked with data from the rest of health, and despite comprehensive data on patient-level transactions, ambulance services have no knowledge of outcomes beyond the hospital door. Thus, there is currently little knowledge of any outcomes for these patients transported by ambulance, even from the level of ED; therefore, strategic questions concerning whether prehospital patient care is optimal, cost-effective or even clinically correct are unanswerable.

Conclusion

Fundamental to ambulance services in 2020 will be the ability to analyse and measure the quality of systems and processes in relation to patient outcomes. Adherence to targets for response times based on averages from other jurisdictions remote in geography, time and design needs to be replaced with carefully analysed linked data using sophisticated statistical techniques, including regression and survival analyses, as well as comprehensive health economic evaluations, in order to allow patient outcomes to be utilised to determine the effectiveness of ambulance practice.

Only when ambulance systems are formally part of health services, overtly providing the prehospital phase of a continuum emergency care, with paramedics assessing patients in a structured, risk-aware form based in clinical reasoning, and with processes, systems and interventions based on proven effectiveness, measured by clinical outcome at later stages in the patient journey, will Australian ambulance services truly have come into the twenty-first century.

References

Abella, B.S. (2013). The importance of cardiopulmonary resuscitation quality. *Current Opinion in Critical Care, 19,* 175–180.

Al-Harbi, N., El-Masri, S., Saddik, B. (2012). An integration of emergency department information and ambulance systems. *Studies in Health Technology Informatics, 180,* 985–989.

Aufderheide, T. P., Sigurdsson, G., Pirrallo, R. G., et al. (2005). Hyperventilation-induced hypotension during cardiopulmonary resuscitation. *Circulation, 109,* 1960–1965.

Australian Commission on Safety and Quality in Health Care, Governance. (2014). http://www.safetyandquality.gov.au/about-us/governance/.

Australian Government Department of Communication. (2012). Broadband availability and quality report. 2012 Dec. http://www.communications.gov.au/__data/assets/pdf_file/0018/212535/Broadband_Availability_and_Quality_Report.pdf.

Bange, R., & van Biljon, W. (2012). Paramedic registration: A progress report. Paramedics Australasia, WA Chapter. 2012 Sept 12. http://www.paramedics.org.au/content/2012/09/Paramedic-Registration-Report-0609.09.pdf.

Blacker, N., Pearson, L., Walker, T. (2009). Redesigning paramedic models of care to meet rural and remote community needs. Paper presented at: 10th National Rural Health Conference. Proceedings of the 10th National Rural Health Conference, editor Gordon Gregory, Cairns Qld, 17–20 May 2009. Canberra: National Rural Health Alliance, 2009. http://ruralhealth.org. au/10thNRHC/10thnrhc.ruralhealth.org.au/papers/docs/Blacker_Natalie_D4.pdf.

Bond, W. F., Deitrick, L. M., Arnold, D. C., Kostenbader, M., Barr, G. C., Kimmel, S. R., Worrilow, C. C. (2004). Using simulation to instruct emergency medicine residents in cognitive forcing strategies. *Academic Medicine, 79,* 438–446.

Brun, P. M., Bessereau, J., Levy, D., Billeres, X., Fournier, N., Kerbaul, F. (2014 Jul). Prehospital ultrasound thoracic examination to improve decision making, triage, and care in blunt trauma. *The American Journal of Emergency Medicine, 32*(7), 817.e1–2. doi: 10.1016/j. ajem.2013.12.063.

Callaham, M. (1997). Quantifying the scanty science of prehospital emergency care. *Annals of Emergency Medicine, 30,* 785–790.

Cheung, W., Middleton, P. M., Davies, S. R., Tummala, S., Thanakrishnan, G., Gullick, J. (2013). A comparison of survival following out-of-hospital cardiac arrest in Sydney, Australia, between 2004–2005 and 2009–2010. *Critical Care and Resuscitation, 15*(3), 241–246.

Cretikos, M., Bellomo, R., Hillman, K., Chen, J., Finfer, S., Flabouris, A. (2008). Respiratory rate: The neglected vital sign. *Medical Journal of Australia, 188*(11), 657–659.

Dean, J. M., Vernon, D. D., Cook, L., Nechodom, P., Reading, J., Suruda, A. (2001). Probabilistic linkage of computerized ambulance and inpatient hospital discharge records: a potential tool for evaluation of emergency medical services. *Annals of Emergency Medicine, 37*(6), 616–626.

Ebinger, M., Fiebach, J. B., Audebert, H. J. (2014a Dec 8). Mobile computed tomography: prehospital diagnosis and treatment of stroke. *Current Opinion of Neurology,* 28(1), 4–9.

Ebinger, M., Winter, B., Wendt, M., Weber, J. E., Waldschmidt, C., Rozanski, M., Kunz, A., Koch, P., Kellner, P. A., Gierhake, D., Villringer, K., Fiebach, J. B., Grittner, U., Hartmann, A., Mackert, B. M., Endres, M., Audebert, H. J., STEMO Consortium. (2014b). Effect of the use of ambulance-based thrombolysis on time to thrombolysis in acute ischemic stroke: a randomized clinical trial. *JAMA, 311*(16), 1622–1631.

Linn, A., Khaw, C., Kildea, H. (2012). Clinical reasoning: A guide to improving teaching and practice. *Australian Family Physician, 41*(1), 18–20.

Middleton, P. M., & Malone, G. (2010). Best clinical practice in the management of the acutely ill or deteriorating patient—A pre-hospital care perspective. Paper presented at: Recognising and responding to clinical deterioration: solutions for safe care. Meeting of the Australian Commission on Safety and Quality in Healthcare; 2010 Nov 8–9: Adelaide, Australia. Accessed at: http://www.safetyandquality.gov.au/wp-content/uploads/2012/11/438781.pdf.

Milander, M. M., Hiscok, P. S., Sanders, A. B., et al. (1995). Chest compression and ventilation rates during cardiopulmonary resuscitation: the effects of audible tone guidance. *Academic Emergency Medicine, 2,* 708–713.

Mundella, W. C., Kennedy, C. C., Szosteka, J. H., Cook, D. A. (2013). Simulation technology for resuscitation training: A systematic review and meta-analysis. *Resuscitation, 84,* 1174–1183.

New South Wales Department of Health. (2008). Submission to the legislative council, general purpose standing committee no.2 the management and operations of the ambulance service of NSW. 2008 July. http://www.ambulance.nsw.gov.au/Media/docs/081020councilreport-83758ed3-d308-46ff-8a4d-0882822581fa-0.pdf.

New South Wales Health: Ambulance Service of New South Wales. Extended Care Paramedics. http://www.ambulance.nsw.gov.au/about-us/Paramedics.html.

O'Hara, R., Johnson, M., Siriwardena, A. N., Weyman, A., Turner, J., Shaw, D., Mortimer, P., Newman, C., Hirst, E., Storey, M., Mason, S., Quinn, T., Shewan, J. (2015). A qualitative study of systemic influences on paramedic decision making: care transitions and patient safety. *Journal of Health Services Research & Policy, 20*(1 Suppl), 45–53.

Paramedics Australasia. (2012). Public risk and public regulation: Response to the Australian health ministers' advisory council consultation paper: Options for the regulation of paramedics. 2012 Sept. http://www.paramedics.org.au/content/2012/09/PA-Submission-on-paramedic-registration-03082012.pdf.

Price, R., Bendall, J. C., Patterson, J. A., Middleton, P. M. (2013). What causes adverse events in prehospital care? A human-factors approach. *Emergency Medicine Journal, 30*(7), 583–588.

Public Health, Seattle and King County. (2014). King County has world's highest survival rate for cardiac arrest. Updated Monday, May 19, 2014. http://www.kingcounty.gov/healthservices/health/news/2014/14051901.aspx.

Rosen, K. R. (2008). The history of medical simulation. *Journal of Critical Care, 23,* 157–166.

Shaban, R., Wyatt Smith, C. M., Cumming, J. J. (2004). Uncertainty, error and risk in human clinical judgment: Introductory theoretical frameworks in paramedic practice. *Australasian Journal of Paramedicine, 2*(1), 1–12.

Thom, O., Keijzers, G., Davies, S., Taylor, D., Knott, J., Middleton, P. (2014). Clinical research priorities in emergency medicine: Results of a consensus meeting and development of a weighting method for assessment of clinical research priorities. *Emergency Medicine Australia, 26*(1), 28–33.

Wayne, D. B., Butter, J., Siddall, V. J., Fudala, M. J., Linquist, L. A., Feinglass, J., Wade, L. D., McGaghie, W. C. (2010). Simulation-based training of internal medicine residents in advanced cardiac life support protocols: A randomized trial. *Teaching and Learning Medicine, 17*(3), 210–216.

Wik, L., Kramer-Johansen, J., Myklebust, H., et al. (2005). Quality of cardiopulmonary resuscitation during out-of-hospital cardiac arrest. JAMA, 293, 299–304.

Prof. Paul Middleton is a specialist in prehospital and emergency medicine, and has worked as part of trauma and helicopter critical care retrieval teams in both the UK and Australia.

Paul is chair of the New South Wales branch of the Australian Resuscitation Council and works as a senior doctor in emergency medicine. He is Clinical Associate Professor in the Discipline of Emergency Medicine at the University of Sydney's Central Clinical School; Conjoint Associate Professor in the Graduate School of Biomedical Engineering and Conjoint Senior Lecturer in the School of Public Health and Community Medicine, both at the University of New South Wales. Paul is the founder and chair of the national cardiac arrest charity, Take Heart Australia.

He is a fellow of the Royal College of Emergency Medicine, the Australasian College for Emergency Medicine, the Royal College of Surgeons of England and the Australian and New Zealand College of Paramedicine, and has published extensive clinical research on non-invasive assessment of illness, prehospital research and clinical trials, patient safety, epidemiology, health economics and critical patient transport.

His former roles include several years as medical director of the Ambulance Service of NSW, founding director of the Ambulance Research Institute and chief medical officer to St John Ambulance, Australia.

Chapter 15
International Perspectives: South African Ambulance Services in 2020

Craig Vincent-Lambert

Introduction: Development of Emergency Medical Services in South Africa

The word "paramedic" literally means "along-side medicine"; a person whose job is to assist and support doctors (The South African Oxford School Dictionary 1998, p. 314). The need for such persons specifically trained to provide immediate care to ill or injured patients in the prehospital setting was identified many years ago during times of war. Injured soldiers on the front line were attended to by "medics" as opposed to doctors and surgeons who were seen as too valuable a commodity to risk placing directly in the front lines.

Early research into survival from traumatic events began to highlight the important link between rapid medical intervention and survival. The concept of the now universally recognised "golden hour" principle began to emerge. The "golden hour" was defined as the first 60 min post injury or insult. Injured patients who received little or no medical intervention during this first hour were noted to be less likely to survive than those who did, even though both may have ultimately ended up in the same receiving facility. This understanding redirected efforts away from simply scooping up the patient and rushing them to hospital toward initiating emergency medical treatment prior to and during transport (Joseph 2002, p. 75).

Whilst the above idea was well supported, there remained insufficient numbers of medical doctors to deploy with each unit. The solution lay in training non-medical personnel and fellow soldiers to provide "primary care" in the field. Initially, this training was rudimentary and focused mainly on the stemming of bleeding, splinting of fractures and simple first aid. However, as time went on, army medics

C. Vincent-Lambert (✉)
Department of Emergency Medical Care, University of Johannesburg,
Cnr Beit and Siemert Street, Doornfontein, Johannesburg 2094, South Africa
e-mail: clambert@uj.ac.za

© Springer International Publishing Switzerland 2015
P. Wankhade, K. Mackway-Jones (eds.), *Ambulance Services,*
DOI 10.1007/978-3-319-18642-9_15

became better trained and their scope of practice subsequently increased. Medics became recognised as a valuable human resource that could render care at the site of injury, stabilise patients and facilitate ongoing care until such time as they could be transported and handed over to a medical doctor at a field hospital or definitive care facility (Vincent-Lambert et al. 2014).

The above concept was imported into the civilian noncombat environment, and it became acknowledged and accepted that ambulance crews were able to do far more than simply rush ill and injured patients to hospital hoping they would be alive on arrival (Caroline 2008, pp. 1.5–1.9).

South African Emergency Medical Services

Prior to 1970, local authorities (town councils) were in the main responsible for the provision of ambulance services in South Africa (SA). Working shifts on an ambulance was in many cases simply seen as an additional and often undesirable "add-on" duty for persons primarily employed in a more recognised role of traffic official and/or firefighter. Although things have changed, the link between firefighting, rescue and emergency care continues, and there are still a number of large "combined" services who render all three functions both locally and abroad (Christopher 2007, pp. 1–12). In contrast to the combined service model, a number of provinces within SA have subsequently removed the responsibility for providing Emergency Medical Services (EMS) away from the local fire/law enforcement departments at municipal level. In these areas, the rendering of EMS now remains the direct responsibility of the provincial government under the umbrella of the National Department of Health (NDoH; Christopher 2007, p. 9).

One criticism of the municipality-based system was that it limited access to EMS for those citizens who lived in rural areas. Unequal access to EMS was further promoted due to the policies of the apartheid government who, prior to 1994 racially segregated and unequally distributed resources in favour of the white population. Non-governmental organisations (NGOs) such as the Order of St. John, Red Cross and the South African First Aid League assisted in servicing calls in many parts of the country with ambulances staffed predominately by volunteers. Levels of care and training varied significantly with many volunteer services only able to provide basic first aid and transport whilst other larger urban centres had access to doctors and nurses for prehospital management of the ill and injured (RSA NDoH 2014).

The subsequent State Health Plan and promulgation of Section 16(b) of the South African Health Act (1974) placed the responsibility for ambulance services with provincial government. With the election of the democratic government in 1994, nine new provinces were established incorporating the former black homelands. This resulted in a dilution of existing available resources.

Prior to 1994, EMS were almost solely rendered by public sector services, either municipal or provincial. The few private providers and NGOs that existed at that time did not routinely render a primary response service; rather, they focused mainly on providing medical cover/standby at planned gatherings and sporting events including performance of inter-facility transfers. Since 1994, service delivery failures of an under-resourced public sector service have resulted in the rapid expansion of private ambulance services who have taken the opportunity to fill service delivery gaps. This resulted in the private sector becoming a significant role player in the South African prehospital environment. Whilst some legislation existed that sought to regulate the establishment and operating of both public and private service providers, it remains poorly enforced.

Education and Training for South Africa Emergency Medical Service

Regardless of which department or sector provides the service, ultimately patients need to be attended to by ambulance crews on the vehicles dispatched to the incidents. The level of care provided by a service is thus determined by the level of education/training and subsequent scope of practice of the staff within their service.

Certain EMS systems, such as that seen in France, offer a doctor-based system with medical doctors responding on emergency vehicles to incidents. In systems like these, prehospital clinical decision-making and medical intervention is at an advanced level and remains the prerogative of the doctor on the vehicle and not the paramedic per se, although doctor-driven paramedics still play an important role in these systems in acting as an assistant to the senior doctor or clinician (Nikkanen et al. 1998, pp. 31, 116–120).

At the other end of the spectrum are EMS systems that operate with ambulance crews that have as little as 3–4 weeks of basic first-aid training. In these systems, clinical decision-making, research and development, formulation of medical protocol and associated clinical governance are also undertaken by medical doctors and not paramedics. In this type of model, paramedics are not usually viewed as independent clinicians or practitioners, and subsequently, their training is more technical in nature, with a strong focus on the following of medical protocol (Ramalanjaona 1998, pp. 31, 766–768).

Three main tiers of emergency care have become generally recognised locally and internationally. These levels are basic life support (BLS), intermediate life support (ILS) and advanced life support (ALS) (Christopher 2007, p. 22). It is also important to acknowledge that the scopes of practice, associated clinical skills and/or procedures that define the boundaries between basic, intermediate and advanced life support remain ill-defined and subject to varied interpretation (Vincent-Lambert et al. 2014). The recent emergence of the emergency care technician (ECT) as a mid-level health worker (MLW) programme for the South African emergency care profession has and continues to generate heated debate as to whether ECT graduates should be considered as advanced life support (ALS) providers.

In SA, EMS education and training historically comprised a number of "short courses" offered alongside formal higher education (HE) diplomas and degrees.

These short courses consisted of a 4-week basic ambulance attendant (BAA) course, a 12-week ambulance emergency assistant (AEA) course and a 9-month critical care assistance (CCA) course (HPCSA 1999a, b, c).

The HE qualifications consisted of a 3-year National Diploma (N. Dip.) and an additional 1-year postgraduate bachelor (B. Tech.) degree.

Three registers historically existed at the Health Professions Council of South Africa (HPCSA) to allow for professional registration. A BLS register for BAA graduates, an ILS register for AEA graduates and an ALS register for CCA and N. Dip. graduates (HPCSA 2011, Online). However, as time went on, a number of problems with this model began to emerge.

During the 1990s and up to the present, the private sector became highly involved in short-course training, specifically in the offering of the 4-week BAA course. BAA training proved to be extremely lucrative with young people across the country being lured to private colleges on a promise of work and then into paying large sums of money for the month-long BAA course. BAAs were being produced in massive numbers that far exceeded that required by the emergency services and NDoH (RSA NDoH 2011). This oversupply did not stop the HPCSA becoming continuously inundated with requests from additional role players throughout the country, all wishing to establish small colleges to offer BAA training.

Although initially compliant at the time of accreditation, many of the short-course colleges simply did not have the capacity or the desire to significantly invest in ongoing quality assurance and current technologies; rather, their main focus became filling their classrooms and offering back-to-back courses in an attempt to generate as much profit as possible (HPCSA 2005, pp. 1–5).

Complaints regarding colleges offering short courses began to surface at the HPCSA. Onsite inspections revealed a sad state of affairs with regard to a lack of quality assurance, insufficient management capacity, equipment deficits, poor teaching and learning conditions and insufficient numbers of qualified staff. With as many as 60 providers being accredited by 2005, quality assurance of emergency care education and training became virtually impossible (HPCSA 2005, pp. 1–5).

The above-mentioned factors naturally resulted in poorly equipped graduates. From an industry perspective, BAAs rapidly became viewed as cheap, semi-skilled labour. It became clear to the NDoH that continued BAA training was not good for the profession. The HPCSA and Professional Board for Emergency Care (PBEC) also realised that BAAs, whilst registered in the category of supervised practice, were being used as independent practitioners. To have BAAs attending to critically ill and injured patients with only a few weeks of training was not seen to be in the interest of the public or the profession (RSA NDoH 2011).

Due to the oversupply of BAAs, thousands who register with the HPCSA are removed from the register each year due to non-payment of annual fees. The main reason cited is that they did not find work as promised by the training providers and they have remained unemployed and therefore simply cannot afford the registration fees (Naidoo 2011).

Despite the fact that anecdotal reports to the contrary are common and aside from all of the associated quality concerns, the short-course system actually failed to produce sufficient numbers of paramedics to meet the needs of the NDoH. Twenty years on, an ALS shortage still exists today with only around 1400 practitioners being on the ALS register (HPCSA 2011, Online; RSA NDoH 2011).

The short courses were never properly re-curriculated and as such continued to operate on more or less the same curriculum since 1990. The academic architecture of the short courses is not South African Qualification Authority (SAQA) compliant. For example, the CCA course contains credits and notional hours in excess of 120, which is the maximum allowed for a short learning programme (SAQA 2011, Online). For these reasons, the short courses lay and continue to lie, outside of the National Qualifications Framework (NQF; RSA NDoH 2011).

Articulation between the short courses and the HE offerings became increasingly difficult as the knowledge gap between these noncredit bearing short courses and the HE qualifications grew ever wider. This created growing amounts of frustration within the service (HPCSA 2005, p. 1).

None of the short-course training providers were ever registered with the Department of Education (DoE) through Umalusi, the Council for Higher Education (CHE), the Department of Labour or Health Workers Seta as training providers for emergency care education. This left the HPCSA as the only Education and Training Quality Assurer (ETQA) for all of these providers.

The professional board for emergency care (PBEC), NDoH and HPCSA sat in an uncomfortable position, whereby the emergency care profession continued to confer professional registration and status to persons who had no formal qualifications and in some cases only a few weeks of training. This was in stark contrast to every other health profession in the country and abroad where professional registration is only possible through the completion of formal HE qualifications.

Finally, the focus of the short-course system was and remains mainly on clinical skills training and not education. The majority of short-course graduates are thus not empowered to adequately function as independent practitioners, provide clinical governance and education, undertake further study within the NQF or participate in research and development. In SA, the emergency care profession has become independent, and the above skills are now expected of all registered professionals.

More Recent Developments

The need to comply with the requirements of the SAQA Act (Act 58 of 1995) provided an opportunity for a review of the entire system of emergency care education and training in SA. The challenge lay in designing a structure which would comply with the needs of the NDoH as well as the emergency care profession. Central to the discussions at that time were important issues of lifelong learning, academic progression, career pathing and placement as well as further professional development. This review and restructuring was undertaken by the PBEC functioning as the standard generating body (SGB). Revision and alignment of the learning outcomes of the existing short courses resulted in the design of a formal 1-year 120 credit NQF level 5 higher certificate and a 2-year 240 credit NQF level 6 diploma in emergency medical care.

The 3-year national diploma and 1-year B. Tech. programme were collapsed and submitted to SAQA in the form of a single 4-year 480 credit NQF level eight professional bachelor of emergency medical care (B. EMC.) degree. The B. EMC. allows for direct articulation into masters and doctoral programmes. On instruction from the HPCSA, HE institutions (HEIs) offering emergency medical care programmes are currently in the process of phasing out the old N. Dip and B. Tech. qualifications and implementing the new 4-year BHS EMC Degree (HPCSA 2009, p. 2). Regulations are also before the Minister of Health, which, if promulgated, will result in the phasing out of short-course training for the emergency care profession.

South African Emergency Medical Service 2020: Future Challenges

The concept of an EMS "system" should be delineated from the concept of "emergency care practitioners" or "providers" who function within a given "system". A number of countries have adopted a *Technician*-based approach to the training of their paramedics. In such systems, training is more technically focused on the following of set protocols and treatment regimes as opposed to definitive diagnosis and clinical decision-making. Although paramedics within such systems can and often do obtain tertiary educational qualifications, it is normally only after achieving their primary emergency medical technician (EMT) training which is very similar to the old South African short-course type format.

HE degrees that are on offer in such countries have commonly been completed part-time or via a limited contact mode and tend to focus more on management, communication, education and humanities with limited or no clinical work nor do they lead to an expanded independent medical scope of practice. These diplomas and degrees cannot be compared to the clinically orientated 4-year full-time bachelor degrees in emergency medical care that are being offered by universities in SA. In such "EMS" systems, the role of clinical decision-making, interrogation, critique and development of medical protocol is still in the main driven by medical doctors and not paramedics.

In SA, a different and unique set-up exists, whereby the emergency care profession has to a large degree developed away from a doctor-driven technician system toward a separate autonomous profession. This is evidenced by the fact that paramedics register with the HPCSA as independent practitioners with prescribing rights as do doctors, and they are answerable to a separate autonomous professional board (Christopher 2007, p. 23).

By implication in SA, the responsibility for clinical decision-making, interrogation, critique and development of prehospital medical protocol and direction is now largely driven and owned by paramedics themselves. Although bachelor, masters

Table 15.1 Details of current emergency care education and training offerings and the number of registrations per category

Registration category	Name of course	Type of course	Alignment with NQF level and credits	[a]Total number per category
Current emergency care education and training				
Basic ambulance assistant	Basic ambulance assistant (BAA)	4-week short course	Not aligned to NQF	54,749
Ambulance emergency assistant (AEA)	Ambulance emergency assistant (AEA)	3-month short course	Not aligned to NQF	8029
Paramedic	Critical care assistant (CCA)	9-month short course	Not aligned to NQF	1563
	National diploma: emergency medical care	3-year qualification	NQF 7; 360 credits	
Emergency care technician (ECT)	National diploma emergency care	2-year qualification	NQF 6; 240 credits	597
Emergency care practitioner (ECP)	Bachelor of technology: emergency medical care	1-year qualification	NQF 7; 120 credits	231
	Bachelors degree: emergency medical care	4-year qualification	NQF 8; 480 credits	

[a] The numbers are as per HPCSA registration statistics—May 2013
NQF National Qualifications Framework

and doctoral qualifications are in place to produce graduates who should be able to assume these roles and responsibilities within the profession. It is early days yet and the extent to which this fledgling autonomous profession is capable of properly fulfilling these important functions is frequently debated.

Further complicating the matter is the fact that the void left when doctors withdrew from operations and clinical governance of prehospital care was never properly filled by degree emergency care practitioners. A few of the larger role-players within the private sector have acknowledged this lack of medical direction and clinical governance as a problem and continue to (within their organisations) make use of medical doctors to fulfil this important role. However, within the public sector, clinical governance and review are all but absent.

It is important to mention that this work should not been seen as a criticism or judgment on either a doctor-driven short-course "technician" or practitioner-based "clinician" system. It is acknowledged that both a technician- and/or clinician-based system can work well if properly implemented. The HPCSA and NDoH in SA have however made it clear that they remain in support of a separate autonomous emergency care profession for prehospital emergency care providers with a three-tiered approach to the provision of emergency care. Having said this, Table 15.1 above shows that most of the current South African EMS workforces have no formal emergency care qualifications and the majority still only a few weeks of training. This being the case, there remains a significant future challenge in creating pathways that will allow for the migration of existing members of the profession who only hold short-course certificates into the NQF.

Conclusion

Prior to 1994, polices of the apartheid government resulted in unequal access to EMS for all citizens. At that time, emergency care was almost solely rendered by public sector services, either municipal or provincial. Since 1994, service delivery failures of an under-resourced public sector system have resulted in the rapid expansion of many private ambulance services.

Education and training for the South African emergency care profession historically took the form of vocational in-house short courses ranging from weeks to months in duration. The intention of the NDoH is to begin to phase out these short courses in favour of formal HE offering which comply with the requirements of SAQA and the NQF.

At present, there are very few degree qualified operational paramedics with the majority of the SA EMS workforce holding no tertiary qualifications. This is set to change as moving into the future; it is envisaged that all persons entering the South African emergency care profession will need to have a recognised HE qualification. The proposed system sees three cadres of provider all holding formal 1-, 2- or 4-year qualifications that reside within the HE band of the NQF. These new providers are:

1. Emergency care assistants (ECAs)
2. Emergency care technicians (ECTs)
3. Emergency care practitioners (ECPs)

The necessary legislation has been promulgated, and registers are already open at the HPCSA to accommodate ECA, ECT and ECP graduates providing them with professional registration and respective scopes of practice.

The concept of a tiered approach with entry level workers, mid-level workers and professional practitioners is neither unique nor foreign to the healthcare professions. Although new in the South African emergency care environment, mid-level worker programmes have already been in place for a while in a number of other countries (Dovlo 2004, pp. 4–9, Online). If the current policies of the NDoH are to remain, mid-level healthcare workers will be introduced in most, if not all of the registered professions including medicine, radiography and environmental health.

References

Caroline, N. (2008). *Emergency care in streets*. London: Jones & Bartlett.
Christopher, L. D. (2007). *An investigation into the non-compliance of advanced life support practitioners with the guidelines and protocols of the professional board for emergency care practitioners*. Masters dissertation, Durban University of Technology, Durban.
Dovlo, D. (2004). *Using mid-level cadres as substitutes for internationally mobile health professionals in Africa. A desk review*. http://www.human-resources-health.com/content/2/1/7. Accessed 20 Jun 2010.

HPCSA (Health Professions Council of South Africa). (1999a). *May 1999: Curriculum for the critical care assistant course*. Doc. 5. Part 1. Pretoria: HPCSA.

HPCSA (Health Professions Council of South Africa). (1999b). *May 1999: Curriculum for the ambulance emergency assistant course*. Doc. 4. Part 1. Pretoria: HPCSA.

HPCSA (Health Professions Council of South Africa). (1999c). *May 1999: Curriculum for the basic ambulance assistant course*. Doc. 2. Part 1. Pretoria: HPCSA.

HPCSA (Health Professions Council of South Africa). (2005). *EC news: Newsletter of the professional board for emergency care*. Pretoria: HPCSA.

HPCSA (Health Professions Council of South Africa). (2009). *EC news: Newsletter of the professional board for emergency care*. Pretoria: HPCSA.

HPCSA (Health Professions Council of South Africa). (2011). Professional board for emergency care. http://www.hpcsa.co.za/board_emergency_registration.php. Accessed 20 Apr 2011.

Joseph, J. (2002). Can the "golden hour" of shock safely be extended to blunt polytrauma patients? *Prehospital and Disaster Medicine, 17*(2), 75.

Naidoo, R. (2011). Untitled. Verbal presentation at the second meeting of the professional board for emergency care held at Idle winds, Hartbeespoort on 25 Feb 2011.

Nikkanen, H. E., Pouges, C., & Jacobs, L. M. (1998). Emergency medicine in France. *Annals of Emergency Medicine, 31*, 116–120.

Ramalanjaona, G. (1998). Emergency medicine in Madagascar. *Annals of Emergency Medicine, 31*, 766–768.

RSA NDoH (Republic of South Africa. National Department of Health). (2011). *Draft national policy on emergency care education and training*. Draft 6. Pretoria: Department of Health.

RSA NDoH (Republic of South Africa. National Department of Health). (2014). *Draft national policy on emergency care education and training*. Draft 7. Pretoria: Department of Health.

SAQA (South African Qualifications Authority). (1995). *A focused study of the development of the national qualifications framework (NQF) with the aim of streamlining its implementation*. Act No. 58 of 1995. Pretoria: Government Printer.

SAQA (South African Qualifications Authority). (2011). *What is a short course? Frequently asked questions*. Number 45. Pretoria: SAQA. http://www.saqa.org.za/show.asp?include!!/span>=about/faq.htm. Accessed 10 Jun 2011.

The South African Oxford School Dictionary. (1998). Oxford: Oxford University Press.

Vincent-Lambert, C., Bezuidenhout, J., & Jansen van Vuuren, M. (2014 May). Are further education opportunities for emergency care technicians needed and do they exist? *African Journal of Health Professions Education, 6(1)·6–9 doi·10 7196/AJHPE.285.*

Dr Craig Vincent-Lambert first graduated with a National Diploma in Ambulance and Emergency Technology from the Technikon Witwatersrand in 1992, since then he has completed a number of additional post graduate degrees and diplomas in the medical, rescue and educational fields. Dr Vincent-Lambert has 25 years of experience in emergency medical care having worked as a South African Fire Fighter/EMT, Medical Rescuer, Operational Advanced Life Support Paramedic and Emergency Care Practitioner. Dr Vincent-Lambert is currently head of the Department of Emergency Medical Care at the University of Johannesburg where he lectures Emergency Medical Care and Medical Rescue. Dr Vincent-Lambert has served on the Professional Board for Emergency Care at the Health Professions Council of South Africa since 2001.

Chapter 16
International Perspectives: Finnish Ambulance Services in 2020

Juha Jormakka and Simo Saikko

Short History of Ambulance Service in Finland

The Helsinki fire department started patient transport services in 1904 but until 1972, there was no medical training for the staff. In 1972, they started the first response training for firefighters. Few occupational colleges started medical technician training in the 1970s, but there were no standards for basic-level staff at that time. The local medical directors chose the kind of education that was good enough for ambulances, so there were major differences in the level of care produced in different areas (Kiira 2012).

The change in education in the 1990s altered the medical technician training to the practical nurse training. The practical nurse students could choose to specialize in ambulance work for the last 6 months of their training. This training was not enough to meet the demands of the field which needed more skills and knowledge base. More ambulances were changing to advanced-level ambulances, and most of the staff members had a nursing degree or some local special training. In the field, there was a need for advanced-level training, and in 1998, the first paramedic training was introduced. Paramedic training is done in universities of applied sciences, and it is the bachelor-level degree training. National Supervisory Authority for Welfare and Health (NSAWH) did not approve paramedics as independent practitioners which needed to include a nursing degree. The paramedic education became a double degree of a bachelor of paramedic and nursing (Kiira 2012).

J. Jormakka (✉) · S. Saikko
Department of Paramedic Nursing, Saimaa University of Applied Sciences, 53850 Lappeenranta, Skinnarillankatu 36, Finland
e-mail: juha.jormakka@saimia.fi

S. Saikko
e-mail: simo.saikko@saimia.fi

© Springer International Publishing Switzerland 2015
P. Wankhade, K. Mackway-Jones (eds.), *Ambulance Services,*
DOI 10.1007/978-3-319-18642-9_16

Helsinki introduced the first medical doctor ambulances in 1972. It was mainly for resuscitations and traffic accidents, but it changed soon to a medical advice unit. Patients were transported by a basic-level ambulance, and the medical doctors were just there for support and advice. Starting in 1990, the first medical helicopter was introduced in Vantaa. It was funded by charity and covered most of the Southern Finland. Helicopters were used in major accidents, high-risk medical situations and for medical advice. Most ambulance staff needed to ask a permission and further advice, before giving any kind of drugs to a patient. This advice was evaluated to be the most important part of the service later on, and it became a best practice for all areas (Kurola 2002). After a few years, other helicopter emergency services were started in different parts of the country, and they covered most of the country. The helicopter emergency medical systems (HEMS) struggled with funding, even though it was a really highly respected service. In 2006, all the HEMS doctors were transferred to health districts, so only the helicopters and the flight crew needed charity funding. In 2010, the helicopters and the staff changed to a new organization called FinnHEMS. FinnHEMS is funded by the government, and there are six helicopters around the country. There are some parts of the country without HEMS coverage as of 2014, but there are plans to get two more helicopters in Finland, so that the whole country would be covered (Nurmi 2014).

The law for emergency medical service changed in 2011, and it has changed our emergency medical systems dramatically. Earlier, every city or municipality could independently choose the kind of emergency medical systems (EMS) that it preferred. Most of Finland was covered by private ambulance services, because they were the cheapest service available. Most medical directors could not get funding for advanced-level ambulance or a higher level of care. Under the new legislation, health districts were responsible for both the whole area and the quality and level of care in that area. There are 20 health districts in Finland and five university hospital areas that coordinate those health districts (Reissell 2011).

Educational Standards in Paramedic Practice (Finland and European Perspective)

The emergency medical direction law in Finland dictates minimum requirements for staff's education in ambulance practice. A basic-level ambulance needs to have the practical nurse training for one staff member and the other one can be a firefighter. An advanced-level ambulance needs a paramedic training for one staff member, and the other staff member can be a firefighter or a practical nurse. There is specialized training for nurses for an advanced-level ambulance. Field directors should have paramedic degree as well as specialized training for field management (Finlex 2011). However, that training is not standardized, and there is no more advanced-level education for paramedics. All the master-level degrees, doctorates and doctor degrees are done from different fields, so there is a need for master's level in para-medic science. The first master-level programmes for paramedics start in 2015 in Finland (Saikko 2014).

The paramedic training in Finland is conducted in eight universities of ap-plied sciences. Those universities work together to improve the quality of trained paramedics. There is a national written examination for paramedics two times in 4 years of training. After 2 years, there is a basic-level written examination, and after 4 years, there is an advanced-level examination. There are also a practical skills evaluation and a simulation evaluation to test graduating paramedics. The idea is that although the universities are independent, there is demand to make sure all paramedics who graduate are evaluated against the same criteria. The criteria for evaluation are evidence based, and all of the tests are approved with all the seven universities. The written examinations are compiled by a workgroup that in-cludes members from all the universities. The examination takes place at the same time throughout Finland six times a year, and it is the same for all the participants. To pass the written test that is conducted online, the students need to score 65 %. Simulations and skills tests are evaluated by the ambulance service staff, who have specialized training for its evaluation and simulation. The evaluation is focused on nontechnical skills and patient safety aspects (Saikko 2014).

The Finnish paramedic education, skill set and knowledge are quite similar when compared to other paramedic educations programmes in Estonia, Poland, Sweden, Germany and the UK. However, despite these similarities, the differences in edu-cational levels are quite considerable. For instance, nurse-based education in Swe-den and Estonia requires short additional training to qualify to work in ambulance. German paramedic training is a high-quality 3 year programme, but it is not an academic degree. In the future, there would be a demand for European standard for paramedic education (Langhelle 2004; Krüger 2009; Saikko 2014).

Quality Factors and Risk Management

All the health districts have to do a risk assessment in their given area. Finland is divided into areas of 1 km^2, and for each area, the risk is evaluated by the number of calls per day, traffic, population, demographics of the area, distance to hospital and a few other different factors. This risk assessment is used as the basis for planning emergency service needed in every area. There are five different risk categories, and all same category areas need to offer similar services. The need for HEMS is also evaluated. The emergency service plan states that if the health district is doing the service by themselves, or if the service is bought from a fire service, or from private companies, then the emergency service plan is done in collaboration with healthcare providers, so that it forms a regional working emergency care body (Reissell 2011).

Future of Ambulance Services: Continuing Education and Professional Development

The standards for staff knowledge and skills are mainly the same, but the evaluation varies between health districts. Most services have written examinations every 2–3 years, and some have simulation tests. A few services do not test the staff at all but arrange simulations to evaluate the need for continuing education. All the areas need to keep statistics of their effectiveness and evaluate those to improve quality. All the mistakes and risky situations are continuously noted down and evaluated. If there are some common mistakes, the annual education is changed to get the staff work better or in more effective ways. The development discussions are conducted yearly, and the staff are directed to the education that they need. Most of the areas do 24-h shifts, and the time between calls is used for skill training and lectures. The health district organizes yearly lectures presenting the updated changes in the system and the protocols (Kosonen 2014).

When the ambulance service is hiring new staff, paramedics are preferred. South Carelia's Social and Health District organises the EMS for the whole area, and 90 % of staff are paramedics (Palviainen 2014). Since the distances are long and the population is rather small, advanced-level units are needed in rural areas for taking care of patients during long-distance transports. A small population means a small number of critical emergencies, so continuing education is highly important (Kosonen 2014).

The ambulance service in Finland is thought to be one part of the emergency department. The idea is that an ambulance crew is working as part of the emergency department. Paramedics can assess patients at home and evaluate if there is a reason to go to a hospital. Some patients are triaged in the ambulance that they can be brought directly to an operating theatre or intensive care unit (ICU), passing the accident and emergencies (A&Es). Some ambulances can use different diagnostic methods like laboratory tests or an ultrasound to evaluate the need for A&E. All the decisions are made in consultation with the emergency department and the patient. Up to 60 % of the patients are not transported to A&E (Kurola 2011; Reissell 2011).

In some health districts, paramedics do short placements yearly in different hospital departments as part of the continuing education. Rotation is done in a different department every year. The normal placement is 2 weeks, and it includes an operating theatre, ICU, A&E and delivery room. Placements are important for knowledge and skills and for later collaboration (Takala 2014).

To conclude, the Finnish health service is changing rapidly to a more centralized service. In most parts of the country, it means longer distances to A&E or delivery room. The ministry of health has made a plan for 2020 to change the ambulance service into a moving emergency department. Patients who can be treated at home would not be transported to hospital anymore. They could get prescription to drugs or medications at home or time could be booked for a health centre, laboratories and X-rays for the next day and patients could be evaluated safely and with low risk. All these require better education for assessing patients, different diagnostic equipment, an electronic documentation system and safe wireless data connections between ambulance and hospital (Kurola 2011; Saarinen 2014). This will help prepare the Finnish ambulance service for the challenges of the twenty-first century.

References

Finlex. (2011). ensihoitoasetus (Finnish law).
Kiira, P. (2012). ELÄMÄÄ hälytysvalmiudessa.
Kosonen, A. (2014). Interview (Senior lecturer, doing research in continuing education, research will be published January 2015).
Krüger, A. (2009). Scandinavian pre-hospital physician-manned emergency medical services— Same concept across borders?
Kurola, J. (2002). Paramedic helicopter emergency service in rural Finland.
Kurola, J. (2011). Jouni Ensihoitopalvelut osana sairaanhoitopiirien toimintaa. *Finnanest, 44,* 116–118.
Langhelle, A. (2004). International EMS systems: The nordic countries 2004.
Nurmi, J. (2014). Interview (Hems MD, Research coordinator).
Palviainen, J. (2014). Interview (South Karelia Social and Health Care District, Head of EMS)
Reissell, E. (2011). On-call social and healthcare services in Finland 2011.
Saarinen, M. (2014). Interview (Prehospital specialist, ministry on health and social services).
Saikko, simo. (2014). Interview (Principal lecturer, Saimaa University of Applied Sciences).
Takala, S. (2014). Interview (Field manager, The Hospital District of Helsinki and Uusimaa, EMS)

Juha Jormakka is a senior lecturer of Paramedic Science in Saimaa University of Applied Sciences in Finland. As a former Special Forces trainer and advanced level paramedic, he is specialized in leadership training, emergency medical service management, international relationships and continuing education. He has master's degree in Health Promotion, and he has done many international exchanges and conferences around the world investigating different Emergency Medical Services. He has published articles in the Finnish paramedic magazine and has presented papers at the ECSSA 2014 Conference in Johannesburg, South Africa, at the Huropel 2012 Conference in Lappeenranta, Finland and the Huropel 2011 Conference in Salford, UK. Juha is currently working on smart ambulance project exploring international links with Russia and the paramedic education development projects in Saimaa University of Applied Sciences.

Simo Saikko is the principal lecturer of Paramedic Science at the Saimaa University of Applied Sciences (SUAS) in Finland. His history includes anaesthesia and intensive care work in several hospitals and also 18 years pre-hospital paramedic work in ambulances. A very important part of his career is related to the Emergency Services College, which is supervised by the Ministry of the Interior. Simo played an important role to start the new academic (bachelor's degree) paramedic education in the 90's in Finland. Simo has written several articles in paramedic magazines and in emergency books. He has professional contacts in Estonia, Sweden, Norway, Germany, Poland and UK. His research interests include simulation pedagogy and the professional skills assessment utilizing simulation technology. Simo is currently developing the new master degree education for paramedics which will start at Saimaa University of Applied Sciences in September 2015. He is working also on international SAEPP Project and the Smart Ambulance Development Project of SUAS.

Index

A
Ambulance service, 3, 4, 17, 33
  improvement of, 37
  in England, 43
  in the UK, 7, 11
  risk in, management of, 32
  role of, 4
  sub-cultures, 10
  twentieth century, 22–24
  understanding of, 7, 8
Austerity, 11, 135, 138
  dealing with, 104
Australian ambulance service, 12, 160, 163, 166
  state of, 164, 165

C
Clinical leadership, 33, 37, 69, 100
Clinical performance indicator care
    bundles, 34, 35
Clinicians, 4, 9, 34, 37, 57–59, 154
Command, 49, 108
  functions of, 111
Commissioning, 5, 9, 51, 52
  ethical ambulance, 52, 53
Communication, 8, 24, 110, 111, 180
Continuing education, 13, 164, 167
  ambulance services, future of, 188
Culture, 5, 9, 65, 69, 82
  ambulance, classification of, 74, 75
  definition of, 10
  in the ambulance service, 70

D
Decision making, 9, 12, 39, 57–59, 113, 180

Demand, 100, 103
  low-acuity, 86
  of emergency, 5
  tick-box, 130

E
Education, 4, 39, 141, 177
Efficiencies, 10, 103, 136, 140
Emergency calls, 6, 99, 107, 139
Emergency demand, 9, 44, 48
Emergency medical care, 180
Emergency medical service (EMS), 83, 177, 180
  in South Africa, development of, 175, 176
Emergency medical systems, 4, 186
Emergency services, 3, 5, 7, 10, 46, 55, 58, 65, 69
Ethical commissioning, 9, 56, 60, 143
Ethnic minority groups, 120

F
Fair, 9, 55, 57, 60, 97
Financial, 9, 11, 31, 150
Funding, 13, 95, 136, 186
  in UK, 22
Future, 4, 12, 13, 103, 158, 160
  challenge in, 181
  models of, 47
  of ambulance services, 188
  perspectives, 11

I
Incident management, 108
Innovation, 8, 26, 95, 96, 135, 138
Interoperability, 10, 108, 109, 115

© Springer International Publishing Switzerland 2015
P. Wankhade, K. Mackway-Jones (eds.), *Ambulance Services,*
DOI 10.1007/978-3-319-18642-9

J

Joint emergency services interoperability
    programme (JESIP), 109, 110, 112,
    114, 115, 144

L

Leadership, 3, 4, 10, 37, 82–84, 166
  definitions of, 81
  of NHS, 68
  role of, 72

M

Modern, 20, 84, 95, 155
  well-equipped, 25
Modernisation, 4, 10, 82, 90

O

Organisations, 4, 5, 10, 70, 181
  NHS, 11, 124

P

Paramedic, 69
Paramedic education, 100, 159, 167, 171,
  185, 187
Paramedicine, 164, 165, 168
Paramedics, 5, 10, 12, 25, 47, 87, 89, 186,
  188
  doctor–driven, 177
  in Australia, 164, 166
  role of, 73, 83
Performance, 4, 5, 67, 100, 103
  definition of, 34
  of clinical, 40
Police, 11, 20, 22, 23, 67, 107
  services of, 109, 111, 114, 115
Prehospital, 3, 9, 11, 34, 83, 136, 139
  development of, 180
  quality improvement in, 36
Prehospital care, 11, 12, 164

Priority setting, 9, 51, 60
  ensuring ethical, 53
Productivity, 84, 86, 87, 95
Professionalism, 24, 70

Q

Quality, 4, 8, 120, 187
  improvement of, 36, 37, 39, 40
  management of, 31–33, 86

R

Reform, 5, 65, 67, 82, 160
Risk, 8, 111, 165, 168, 169
  in ambulance services, management of, 32
  practice of, 31
  quality factors and, 187
Roles, 25, 69, 71, 97, 181

S

Science, 7, 159, 185, 187
Skills, 10, 11, 26, 100, 152, 171, 187
  extending roles and, of ambulance, 71, 72
Structure, 3, 10, 13, 33, 108, 179
  issues of, 157
Systems, 68, 103, 155, 177
  computer-aided, 26
  quality of, 12

T

Technology, 66, 88, 159
Transport, 3, 10, 17, 24, 48, 84, 138, 188
  of patient, 21, 26, 140, 158, 159, 169

U

Urgent Care, 4, 7, 47, 85, 103

V

Vision 2020, 166, 172

Printed by Printforce, the Netherlands